THE **COMPLETE** GUIDE TO

Judy DiFiore

POSTNATAL FITNESS

3rd Edition

A & C Black · London

Published by A&C Black Publishers Ltd
36 Soho Square, London W1D 3QY
www.acblack.com

Third edition 2010
Second edition 2003
First edition 1998

Copyright © 2010, 2003, 1998 Judy DiFiore

ISBN 978 1 4081 2455 0

A CIP catalogue record for this book is available from the British Library.

Acknowledgements
Cover photograph © Shutterstock
Inside photographs © Grant Pritchard
Illustrations by Jeff Edwards

This book is produced using paper that is made from wood grown in managed, sustainable forests. It is natural, renewable and recyclable. The logging and manufacturing processes conform to the environmental regulations of the country of origin.

Typeset in 10.5 on 12pt Baskerville BE Regular by Palimpsest Book Production Limited, Falkirk, Stirlingshire.

Printed and bound in Croatia by Zrinski

ACKNOWLEDGEMENTS

My fascination with the amazing journey of the pregnant body began in 1988 when, as a tutor for London Central YMCA (as they were then) I became involved in the development of the first ante/postnatal teacher training course of its kind. Pregnant with my first son, and with no idea of what lay ahead, I worked alongside three women's health physiotherapists, Molly Jennings, Sue Lewis and Gillian Fletcher, whose enthusiasm and dedication to ante/postnatal exercise inspired me to specialise in this field.

Twenty-two years on I continue to develop my knowledge and have been fortunate to attend presentations by key international speakers, both at home and abroad, whose research enables us to have a better understanding of the effects of pregnancy and childbirth on the remarkable female body.

Through my association with the Guild of Pregnancy and Postnatal Exercise Instructors, I have had the pleasure of working alongside fellow ante/postnatal exercise specialist Moira Clark. A real expert in her field, Moira has been an invaluable sounding board for thoughts and ideas on how new research can be best applied to the exercise environment. I would like to thank her for her meticulous proofreading of this book, tireless feedback and positive, constructive comments. I would also like to thank women's health physiotherapists Daphne Sidney and Pauline Walsh for their support and comprehensive feedback over the last two years, and Sue Lewis and Jacqui Schirmer for helping me with the numerous queries that arose.

A special mention to my sister Jill Richardson for her excellent proofreading skills and for her support and encouragement when the going got tough – which it did!

I could not have written this without the hands-on experience of real postnatal teaching, so I would like to thank all my postnatal mums and their babies over the last 20 years, for helping me learn and develop from them and for making my job so rewarding.

Above all, I would like to thank my wonderful husband, Mike, for his tolerance while I put my life on hold to complete this edition!

This book is dedicated to the memory of
my wonderful dad:
may his spirit live forever!

CONTENTS

INTRODUCTION

It takes nine months for a woman to develop and nurture a new life and her body must undergo many complex and amazing changes. So why is it that the minute baby is born, women are expected to get their pre-pregnancy shape back and be a supermum?

Much of the pressure is put on women by themselves but if media images were more realistic perhaps women would give themselves and their bodies longer to recover. Women should be encouraged to respect their post-baby bodies for the wonderful gift of life and celebrate motherhood – but that doesn't mean becoming a couch potato!

Instructors have a responsibility to 'save women from themselves' by guiding and advising them how to do this sensibly and safely. Rushing back to exercise and participating in unsuitable activities will increase the risk of long-term physical problems. Return to fitness and regular weight should be viewed as a long-term goal for health-related fitness.

The fact that you are reading this suggests you are interested in providing the correct advice – but what about instructors who don't know or don't have the inclination to find out? The inclusion of postnatal women in mainstream classes is a regular occurrence and instructors teaching in such settings have a responsibility to provide safe alternatives, rather than just advising women to 'take it easy'. Unconscious incompetence is very dangerous!

It isn't just a matter of her starting where she left off and resuming her pre-pregnancy training programme; major changes have occurred in the structural support systems of a postnatal woman and her body continues to be vulnerable, particularly if breastfeeding. A postnatal programme should focus on the journey back to the pre-pregnancy body with particular consideration for poor lumbopelvic stability, reduced joint stability and postural changes. Re-education of incorrect muscle patterns and correction of muscle imbalances should be addressed before fitness can be progressed and spending time dealing with these issues should be the first priority. Women also need guidelines for managing their bodies in everyday activities and instructors should incorporate this advice into their teaching as much as possible.

Women should not commence formal exercise until they have completed a satisfactory postnatal check-up, which is normally conducted around six weeks after delivery; those who had caesarean deliveries are recommended to wait a couple of weeks longer.

ABOUT THE GUIDE

The Complete Guide to Postnatal Fitness was written in response to the demand for more detailed information on the subject from group fitness instructors and personal trainers.

This third edition has been completely revised and updated and is presented at a higher level than the previous two. It is full of the latest research available, with all references cited for further reading if desired. Some topics lack scientific evidence and this has been discussed where relevant. In such cases, the recommendations have been based on a sound knowledge of the anatomical and physiological implications of pregnancy and delivery, together with more than 22 years' experience of teaching postnatal fitness.

As always, the minute a book goes to print new research is released so the onus must be on the instructor to stay up to date through further reading and training. Science never stands still – keep learning and exploring this field of fitness as there is always more to learn!

HOW TO USE THE GUIDE

Whilst it is hoped you will read the guide from cover to cover, it is also intended as an essential resource for you to dip in and out of as required. With this in mind, the chapters are all self-contained and cross-referenced as necessary.

Part One looks at the anatomical and physiological implications of pregnancy and delivery, how these will affect the return to exercise in the postnatal period, and how exercise can help the body to recover quicker. It is vital that this section is read and fully understood before teaching postnatal women, and referral back to it is recommended from time to time.

Part Two is all about exercise. It looks at cardiovascular and resistance training methods and a range of specific fitness sessions in terms of their suitability during the postnatal period. It also contains a fully detailed programme of appropriate postnatal exercises.

Part Three is concerned with planning, management, teaching and evaluation of a specific postnatal exercise session and the strategies involved in its success.

For ease of writing the early postnatal period is defined as birth to six weeks and the extended postnatal period is anything after that time.

BENEFITS OF POSTNATAL EXERCISE

Posture
- Improved lumbopelvic stability
- Correction of pregnancy stance
- Strengthening muscles that have lengthened
- Lengthening muscles that have shortened
- Redressing muscular imbalance
- Awareness of posture while feeding/lifting/carrying
- Awareness of back, abdominal and pelvic care

Functional capacity
- Improved lumbopelvic stability
- Increased strength and endurance for activities of daily living
- Improved aerobic fitness
- Increased ability to deal with the everyday demands of a new baby
- Reduced fatigue – increased energy

General health
- Boosted immune system
- Improved sleep quality
- Improved circulation and healing
- Improved digestion

Body composition
- Increased muscle mass
- Increased metabolic rate
- Increased calorific burning
- Increased fat loss

Social and emotional well-being

- Increased production of endorphins
- Enhanced self-image and self-confidence
- Personal satisfaction and achievement
- Personal identification
- Increased social interaction

RISKS OF POSTNATAL EXERCISE

- Fatigue and exhaustion
- Injury from reduced joint stability
- Injury from poor lumbopelvic stability
- Injury from inappropriate exercises or technique

Contraindications to exercise

- Joint or pelvic girdle pain
- Inadequate healing, discomfort
- Excessive fatigue
- Gross separation of rectus abdominis

STRUCTURE AND FORM

THE PELVIS

Structure of the pelvis

The pelvis is made up of four bones: two hip bones, plus the sacrum and the coccyx. Each hip bone is made up of three fused bones: ilium, ischium and pubis. The acetabulum, the deep socket for the head of the femur, is formed by the unification of all three bones.

- The **ilium** is the large wing-shaped part of the pelvis providing a broad surface area for muscle attachment. The upper border, the iliac crest, can be felt when the hands are placed on the hips. The bony points at each end of the iliac crest can be felt at the front of the pelvis, as the anterior superior iliac spines (ASIS), and at the back, as the posterior superior iliac spines (PSIS). These are useful landmarks when checking correct postural alignment as they should be approximately at the same level.
- The **ischium** is the thick, lower part of the pelvis leading down to the ischial tuberosities, commonly referred to as the 'sit bones'.
- The **pubis** is at the front of the pelvis where the two pubic bones join to form the symphysis pubis at the top and the pubic arch underneath.
- The **sacrum** is a triangular-shaped bone made up of five fused vertebrae. It is joined to the ilium by the sacroiliac joints, which are positioned on either side of the sacrum.
- The **coccyx** consists of four fused vertebrae that are joined to the sacrum at the sacrococcygeal joint.

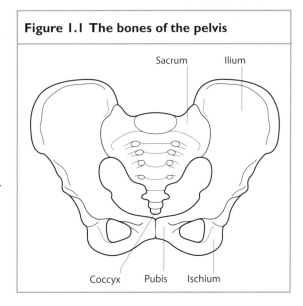

Figure 1.1 The bones of the pelvis

Sacrum   Ilium

Coccyx   Pubis   Ischium

The joints of the pelvis

The pelvis is made of two halves that join at the front at the symphysis pubis and at the back at the sacroiliac joints.

- The **symphysis pubis** (SP) is situated at the front of the pelvis where the two pubic bones meet. Separated by a pad of cartilage resembling a vertebral disc, the joint is approximately 4mm wide and has minimal movement, except in pregnancy.
- The **sacroiliac joints** (SIJ) join the spine to the pelvis (one on each side) between the ilium and the sacrum. The strongest joints in the body, they transmit forces from the upper body and ground reaction forces from the lower extremities. The SIJ allow limited backward and forward movement during flexion

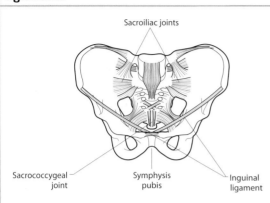

Figure 1.2 Joints of the pelvis showing ligaments

Sacroiliac joints

Sacrococcygeal joint

Symphysis pubis

Inguinal ligament

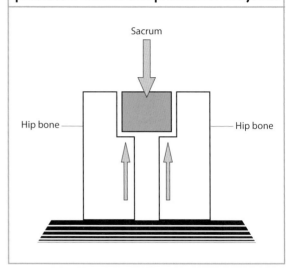

Figure 1.3 Form closure of the pelvis provides a natural compression of the joints

Sacrum

Hip bone

Hip bone

and extension of the trunk. During gait the joints lock alternately to allow transmission of body weight from the sacrum to the hip bone. They are synovial (gliding) joints, held together by both anterior and posterior ligaments. By 30 years of age the SIJ lose their synovial quality and become more cartilaginous (Mercer 2009).

- The **sacrococcygeal joint**, situated between the sacrum and the coccyx, is worth a mention as it allows a small amount of flexion and extension of the coccyx. This is necessary during labour to increase the size of the pelvic outlet.

Form and force closure

These are mechanisms to prevent excessive movement at a joint. Form closure relates to the structure of the joints, bones and ligaments; force closure is the activation of muscles and fascia, together providing stability for a joint. These mechanisms are particularly relevant to pelvic stability during pregnancy.

Form closure of the pelvis

The structure of the SIJ provides excellent form closure. The triangular-shaped sacrum is wedged in between the two hip bones, securing its posi-

tion, and the irregular shape and coarse texture of the bony surfaces interlock with each other to help close the joint. The inner surface of the joint is covered in smooth cartilage to promote glide. Very strong ligaments provide additional support.

The SP has less form closure as the joint is relatively flat. As a cartilaginous joint, it has no synovial capsule – the two ends have 'grown together' and are held together by fibrocartilage. Lee (2007 (i)) suggests it is more vulnerable to shearing forces than the SIJ. Its stability is dependent on the correct alignment of the SIJ and it relies more on the muscular system for support.

Force closure of the pelvis

As discussed above, the structure of the pelvis provides a natural compression of the joints but a degree of mobility is necessary to allow movement to occur. Force closure is the action of muscles around the joints to increase compression at the moment of loading. The amount of force closure required depends on the individual's

Figure 1.4 Force closure of the pelvis is provided by the muscles surrounding the joint

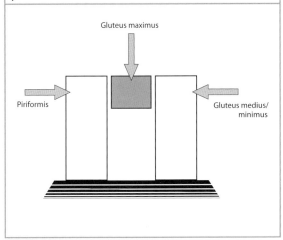

form closure and the size of the load (Lee 2007 (ii)).

Numerous muscles attach onto the pelvis to provide increased lumbopelvic stability from all aspects, but the SP and SIJ are not so well served. At the SP, for example, no muscles actually cross the joint; the closest muscular support comes from fibres of the adductor longus and the abdominal aponeurosis that feed into the anterior ligament, which then crosses the joint. At the SIJ the piriformis is the only muscle to cross it. A deep lateral rotator of the hip, the piriformis originates from the anterior side of the sacrum and attaches to the greater trochanter of the femur. The implications for this are discussed later in this chapter.

Effects of pregnancy on form and force closure

Increased joint laxity during pregnancy has major implications for pelvic stability due to its effects on form closure. Relaxin (*see* below) specifically targets the pelvic ligaments and increases the size of the pelvic outlet in preparation for a vaginal delivery. Lax ligaments reduce joint support,

increase range of movement and reduce form closure. Weight gain and pressure from the baby exacerbate the situation. Jain & Sternberg (2005) suggest there is frequently up to 1cm separation of SP during pregnancy and labour.

With the lack of ligamentous support the muscular system is required to step in and assist with the stabilising role and the body relies on this much more during pregnancy. The effects of this are discussed in chapter 2.

Pelvic girdle pain (PGP)

This is an umbrella term for all problems relating to the pelvis that may occur separately or in conjunction with low back pain. It is a common complaint for women during pregnancy, causing considerable disability and distress (Gutke et al. 2006) and is believed to occur in one in five pregnant women (ACPWH 2007). PGP is associated with changes to form and force closure mechanisms during pregnancy and is discussed in chapter 6.

Relaxin

What is relaxin?

Relaxin is a hormone produced in both pregnant and non-pregnant women (Bani 1997). In non-pregnant women and those in the early stages of pregnancy it is produced by the corpus luteum, which is a yellow mass left behind in the ovaries following ovulation. In the second trimester the placenta and the decidua take over production. Relaxin levels peak during the first trimester, then fall approximately 20 per cent for the remainder of the pregnancy. Production ceases with delivery of the placenta and resumes with the recommencement of the menstrual cycle. Levels are higher in second and subsequent pregnancies and in women carrying more than one baby.

What effects do increased levels of relaxin have on the body during pregnancy?

The most significant pregnancy changes occur in the collagen component of connective tissue. As one of the principal proteins of connective tissue, collagen provides strength and resistance to pulling forces and is found in bone, cartilage, tendons and ligaments. Elastin, as its name suggests, gives elastic strength to connective tissue. Increased levels of relaxin affect the remodelling structure of collagen by increasing elasticity and reducing strength. Joint stability is particularly affected, as ligaments are unable to provide the same degree of support as before.

The degree of change is variable among women and not just dependent on the level of circulating relaxin (Marnoch et al. 2003). Collagen type, which is genetically determined, is a key factor – women with a higher proportion of weaker collagen type, e.g. hypermobile women, will be more at risk during this time. Increased ligament elasticity allows the pelvic joints a greater range of movement and, together with the forward tilt of the sacrum, provides a natural adaptation to accommodate the growing baby. Depending on the position adopted, the pelvic outlet may increase by as much as 28 per cent during delivery.

Which joints are most at risk?

While all joints will be affected to some degree, it is the pelvis that is mostly at risk due to the number of relaxin receptor sites located there. The reduction in form and force closure, together with the progressive pressure exerted by the growing baby, makes the pelvic joints particularly vulnerable. However, during exercise all joints are susceptible to injury; particular care should be taken to ensure that the alignment of ankles, knees, hips, wrists, elbows and shoulders is not compromised by heavy/repetitive loads or momentum.

Are muscles affected by relaxin?

Connective tissue surrounds bundles of muscle fibres that merge together and it extends beyond the muscle to form the tough, inelastic tendon. During pregnancy the proportion of weaker collagen affords a greater range of movement for the muscle and its attachments. The abdominal musculature undergoes the greatest change as it stretches to allow the uterus to grow. The pelvic floor muscles endure increasing pressure during pregnancy and are stretched considerably during delivery. This adaptation severely reduces the support previously given by these muscles and has major implications for muscle function and support (*see* chapters 3 and 4).

What happens to relaxin after delivery?

Production of relaxin ceases on delivery of the placenta. However, connective tissue changes that have occurred will continue until new tissue has been re-formed in the absence of relaxin. Foti et al. (2000) suggest laxity may continue for six months postpartum. Reduced joint stability is a major consideration when exercising postnatally, as the body continues to be vulnerable during this time.

Do the joints regain their stability?

If the joints have been overextended during pregnancy, the ligaments may not provide sufficient stabilisation. However, if appropriate care has been taken, the ligaments should return to their pre-pregnancy inelastic state once the lingering effects of relaxin have left the body. The absence of pressure from the baby greatly reduces the risks to the pelvis, but while the increased range of movement is still evident, the pelvis should be treated with much respect (*see* chapter 2).

Breastfeeding women may find increased joint laxity continues until feeding stops. Prolactin's suppressive effects on oestrogen production contributes to lack of strength and stiffness in connective tissue and this may prolong joint instability (Calleja-Agius 2009). Breastfeeding women, therefore, may feel weaker for longer. Walsh (2008) suggests joint stability improves three months after breast-feeding stops.

Relaxin and postnatal exercise

The lingering effects of relaxin are one of the main risk factors for postnatal exercise. The following areas should be considered.

Range of movement

Care should be taken to protect the joints against injury by ensuring all movements are performed within the normal range of the joint. Speed is an important consideration as fast, particularly long-levered, movements will increase momentum and could easily result in overextension of the joint. Activities such as Tai-Bo, kick boxing and karate carry an additional risk as the fast, jerky movements may encourage joint locking or twisting. Studio resistance classes should be avoided by inexperienced participants; skilled individuals may return to the activity once lumbopelvic stability has been regained (*see* chapter 2). Range of movement should be considered with some yoga postures to avoid overextending unstable joints. While salsa moves may encourage excessive lumbopelvic movements they may help release thoracic tension from gripping spinal extensors (*see* page 20). Participation in this type of class may be suitable for postnatal women once a degree of lumbopelvic stability has been recovered.

Alignment and technique

All movements should be performed with correct body alignment with close attention to technical detail. Locking out, or hyperextension, of elbows and knees should be avoided at all times. Neutral spine (*see* page 29) should be maintained throughout and a tall upright stance adopted where appropriate. Movements involving repetitive joint actions, such as the stepper or cross-trainer, should be monitored for duration, with adjustments made for range of movement to avoid misalignment of the pelvis. Gym and studio cycling may cause discomfort in the SP/SIJ if the seat height is not set correctly (*see* chapters 9 and 11). Increased quadriceps angle (Q angle) of the femur will compromise knee alignment during all weight-bearing activities.

Flexibility work

Stretching to increase flexibility should be avoided until 16–20 weeks after the baby is born, or longer if breastfeeding continues. Attempting to take a stretch further than joint range normally permits could severely compromise joint stability, and the overextension of ligaments may be permanent. Stretching to *maintain muscle length* is strongly recommended and crucial for rebalancing posture. Comfortable stretch positions can be held for longer (up to 30 sec) but no attempt should be made to try to stretch further. Some yoga postures may encourage overextension, particularly if they are held for some time. Care should be taken when participating in this type of activity in the first few months after delivery and instructors should provide alternative postures where appropriate.

High-impact activities

These should be avoided for the first few months to allow sufficient time for joint and lumbopelvic stability recovery. Lactating breasts will feel uncomfortable and place further stress on their delicate support structures. Pressure on the joints is increased twofold with high-impact activities, which put particular strain on the ankles, knees, pelvis and spine. Running is only appropriate if a low-impact stride is practised, minimising vertical action and absorbing the shock through a heel-toe action. Gait should be closely observed for signs of incorrect patterning (*see* chapter 9). Experienced runners may need to review their technique.

Resistance training

This relates to the use of resistance equipment in the gym or a studio resistance class. Experienced lifters who continued to train during pregnancy should recommence at the same resistance they were lifting prior to delivery. If resistance training was not undertaken during pregnancy they should recommence at 70 per cent of their pre-pregnancy load. A heavy weight pulling on an unstable joint, working from an unstable base, increases the risk of joint injury and compromises postural alignment. It is for this reason that it is not advisable for newcomers to exercise with weights initially. Correct recruitment of the stabilising muscles must be established before adding resistance (*see* chapter 2). Clear teaching of technique is important together with guidelines for getting into and out of position on equipment. Close observation and correction by the instructor is essential.

THE SPINE

Structure of the spine

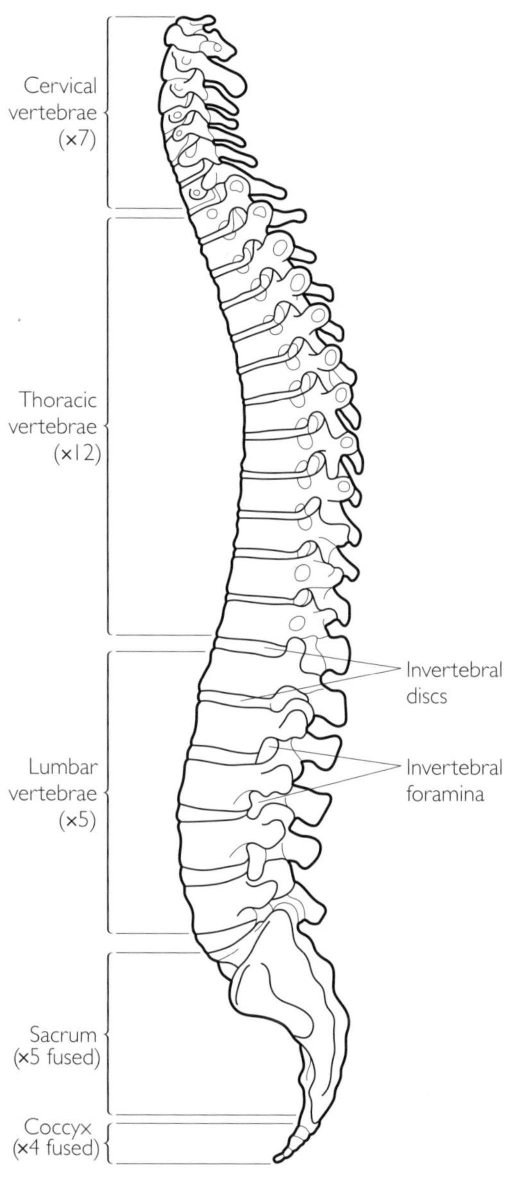

The vertebral column is made up of 33 bones: 24 separate vertebrae, five vertebrae fused to form the sacrum, and another four fused to form the coccyx. The spine has enormous strength, but since it is made up of small sections it is also very flexible and this allows a large range of movement. The vertebrae are separated by intervertebral discs of fibrocartilage, which cushion the vertebrae against jarring and help to keep the spine upright. The curves of the spine are vital for shock absorption: without them the

Figure 1.5 Structure of the spine

Cervical vertebrae (×7)

Thoracic vertebrae (×12)

Lumbar vertebrae (×5)

Invertebral discs

Invertebral foramina

Sacrum (×5 fused)

Coccyx (×4 fused)

base of the brain would receive the full impact when jumping. The spine is dependent on ligaments as well as muscles for its stability.

Correct spinal alignment

Neutral spine is the optimal positioning of the spinal curves, i.e. the inward curve (lordosis) of the cervical and lumbar spine and the outward curve (kyphosis) of the thoracic spine. In this position, pressure is equally distributed along the length of the spine, enabling absorption of impact while minimising stress on bone and soft tissue. When the spine is correctly balanced, body weight is supported primarily through the bones. Only a very small amount of muscular contraction is needed, from the abdominals and spinal extensors, to maintain equilibrium. Recent research suggests correct upright spinal alignment is the No. 1 endurance exercise for the deep stabilising muscles (Richardson 2008, O'Dwyer 2009) and this position should be adopted whenever possible.

The benefits of neutral spine include:
- Improved body mechanics and neuromuscular efficiency
- Reduction and/or elimination of pain
- Prevention of injury
- Improved circulation
- Improved body shape and a more slender appearance
- Increased flexibility
- Improved co-ordination and sense of balance
- Optimal breathing
- Release of pent-up tensions

Figure 1.6 Finding neutral pelvis: a) placement of the hands, b) anterior pelvic tilt, c) posterior pelvic tilt, d) neutral pelvis

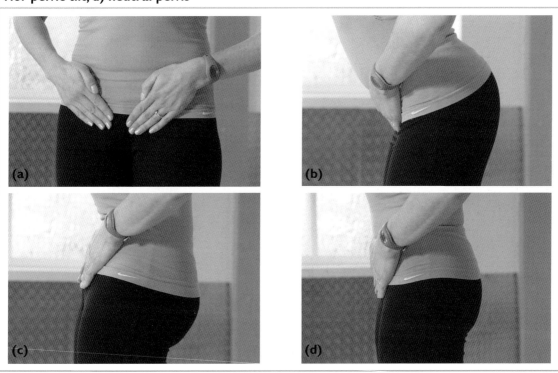

(a)

(b)

(c)

(d)

Neutral pelvis

One of the key aspects of correct spinal alignment relates to the position of the pelvis. Incorrect placement of the pelvis, i.e. anterior or posterior tilt, will have compensatory effects on the spinal curves.

Finding neutral pelvis

Stand with feet hip-width apart and knees soft. Place the heel of your hands on the prominent bones at the front of your pelvis (ASIS) and fingertips on your pubic bone. Tilt the top of the pelvis forwards so that your fingertips move downwards and the natural curvature in your back has increased (anterior pelvic tilt). Now tilt your pelvis the opposite way by lifting your pubic bone upwards so that your fingertips move upwards (posterior pelvic tilt). Feel your back straightening as the natural curvature disappears. Now find a position midway between these two extremes where your fingertips and heel of hands are on the same vertical plane. Buttocks and front of thighs should be relaxed. This is the correct positioning of the pelvis.

> **Important!**
>
> Neutral spine is the 'ideal' position and is used as an alignment reference throughout the book. Maintaining this 'ideal' will be challenging for most postnatal women and variations may be necessary to accommodate individual differences. The role of the instructor is to provide guidance on the journey back to the 'ideal' position.

Effects of pregnancy on spinal alignment

- Increased elasticity of the spinal and pelvic ligaments
- Forward pull of the abdomen as the uterus grows out of the pelvis and into the abdominal cavity
- Reduced likelihood of maintaining neutral pelvis due to increased load
- Inability of overstretched abdominal muscles to support the spine and maintain correct pelvic tilt
- Increased size and weight of the breasts

Compensatory changes occurring in spinal alignment are discussed later in this chapter.

Posture

Posture is strongly influenced by habit and controlled by our own kinesthetic awareness of what 'feels right' – good or bad. It is not a static position – the body is constantly moving and alignment is continually being challenged. Posture relates to the position of the spine and is governed by the strength and suppleness of opposing muscles.

Correct standing posture

- Stand, with the feet hip-width apart (underneath ASIS).
- Spread weight equally between both feet.
- Distribute weight evenly between big toe, little toe and heel.
- Soften the knees and align them over the ankles.
- Find your neutral pelvis (*see* above).
- Slide your shoulders down and relax your elbows.
- Lengthen your tailbone towards the floor, keeping your buttocks relaxed.
- Extend your spine upwards.
- Lengthen the neck, keeping the chin parallel to the floor.
- Look straight ahead.

Why is correct posture so important?

When the body is misaligned it has to work harder to maintain an upright stance. Muscles not designed to support the body are recruited to take up the slack and become overly tight. In addition to placing extra strain on the joints

Figure 1.7 a) correct posture, b) lordotic posture, c) swayback posture

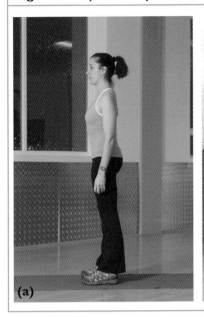 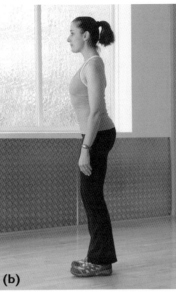 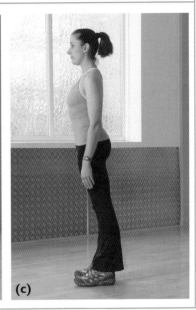

(a) (b) (c)

and their support structures, tight muscles will decrease range of movement and pull the body out of alignment. If that's not enough, overly lax muscles tire easily in the attempt to counter-balance the forces and the body begins to sag. Distortion of the spinal curves increases the degree of compression on the vertebrae and intervertebral discs and decreases blood flow. This is exactly what happens during pregnancy! (*See* chapter 2 for further discussion on stabil-ising muscles.)

Factors affecting postnatal posture

- Pre-pregnancy postural imbalances
- Postural changes occurring during pregnancy
- Size of the baby – antenatal and postnatal
- Age of the baby
- Amount of weight gain
- Level of fitness – before, during and after pregnancy
- Degree of body awareness

COMMON MUSCULOSKELETAL CHANGES OF PREGNANCY

There is no 'normal' pregnancy posture; the adaptations that occur may be an exaggeration of existing postural imbalances and this high-lights the need for individual observation and programming. There are, however, a variety of common postural adjustments which often begin in the lumbar spine and induce compensatory adjustments in the thoracic and cervical spine.

Lumbar

The forward pull of the abdomen may displace the pelvis forwards, with or without a posterior tilt, as seen in swayback postures. To compensate for the forward shift and maintain balance, the upper body sways backwards, creating a high lumbar lordosis. Alternatively, the loss of tone in rectus abdominis (RA) reduces the ability to

maintain correct pelvic alignment and may result in an anterior tilt. Carrying baby on one hip pulls the lumbar spine into lateral flexion as the pelvis tilts to the side. The following adaptations should be taken into account:
- Shortening and tightening of lumbar extensors
- Lengthening and tightening of hamstrings with anterior tilt, or shortening and tightening with posterior tilt
- Shortening and tightening of hip flexors with anterior tilt, or lengthening and weakening with posterior tilt
- Lengthening and weakening of gluteus maximus
- Lengthening and weakening of RA, transversus abdominis (TrA) and external/internal obliques (EO/IO)

Implications for exercise:
- Reduced range of movement in lumbar spine and anterior hip
- Reduced ability to maintain correct pelvic alignment
- Reduced lumbopelvic stability
- Overactive and dominant hamstrings

Thoracic

Flaring of the lower ribcage in the third trimester and the rise of the uterus into the upper abdominal cavity reduce thoracic mobility. Postnatally, the dramatic increase in breast size, if breast feeding, the adoption of poor feeding positions and the repetitive forward bending with 24/7 baby care further magnify the problem. The following adaptations should be taken into account:
- Shortening and tightening of pectorals and upper trapezius
- Resulting medial rotation of humerus
- Corresponding lengthening and tightening in rhomboids and mid-trapezius

- Lengthening and weakening of lower trapezius, posterior rotator cuff and serratus anterior

Implications for exercise:
- Reduced range of movement in thoracic spine
- Reduced range of movement in shoulder joint
- Faulty alignment of all muscles crossing the shoulder joint
- Increased risk of tendon or nerve impingement

Cervical

Increased cervical lordosis occurs as a compensatory effect of increased thoracic kyphosis. The eyes will always seek horizontal, so this is an adjustment made by the brain to ensure effective vision. Also known as 'forward head position', it is characterised by chin poke. The following adaptations should be taken into account:
- Shortening and tightening in neck extensors
- Corresponding lengthening and weakening of neck flexors

Implications for exercise:
- Reduced range of movement in the neck and shoulder
- Increased risk of nerve impingement

Compensatory changes in the hip and lower extremities

Changes in pelvic alignment reduce the lateral support available from gluteus medius. This, together with lengthened and weakened EO, increases lateral sway and reduces control of pelvic movements. Increased activation of other muscles becomes essential to provide the necessary support and this has implications for the hip, knee and ankle.

Shortening and tightening of the deep lateral hip rotators – in particular piriformis – may occur in an attempt to secure the lax SIJ. The sciatic nerve runs underneath piriformis (and sometimes through it) so this has implications for sciatic nerve compression. Overactivity in these muscles draws the head of the femur to the front of the acetabulum with potential for hip or groin pain (Lee 2007 (iii)). Lateral rotation of the hip also increases tension in the iliotibial band and vastus lateralis. This changes the Q angle of the knee and may cause pain.

What is the Q angle of the knee?

This relates to the ability of the patella to track in the patello-femoral groove and is determined by the quadriceps' angle of pull. Muscular balance on the lateral and medial sides of the knee will help maintain its integrity. Deviations may compromise the biomechanics of the knee joint.

On the medial side of the thigh, compensatory lengthening and tightening may occur in the adductors (longus in particular) as they attach onto the pubis and attempt to hold onto the lax SP. Vastus medialis weakens with the change in Q angle. Continuing down to the feet, the wider stance and laterally rotated hips may cause toeing out. Lax ligaments result in dropped arches in the feet and eversion of the ankle. As the centre of gravity moves further forwards during pregnancy, activity in the calves increases to maintain balance; this leads to their shortening and tightening and increases the likelihood of cramps. Corresponding lengthening and weakening occurs in tibialis anterior. Toeing out may also change the angle of pull on the calves, with increased risk of nerve compression.

Implications for exercise:
- Reduced pelvic stability from gluteus medius and EO, which together with tight thoracic spine increases lateral sway during gait
- Reduced range of movement around the hip
- Reduced forces through the quadriceps group during knee extension
- Increased vulnerability of the knee joint
- Poor foot action and reduced absorption of ground reaction forces

Postural retraining

This is crucial to redress the balance of pregnancy and postnatal-induced changes. Individuals will present with varying degrees of misalignment and the role of the instructor is to work towards restoring 'ideal' posture. Postnatal women need to relearn recruitment of the deep stabilisers and rebalance alignment through strength and stretch in opposing muscles.

A postnatal programme should not only address the above changes but also focus on functional movements that train the body to perform everyday tasks in a safe, appropriate way. A baby makes many new and repetitive demands on the body, i.e. getting in and out of bed for unsociable feeds, manoeuvring car seats, and repeated bending, lifting and carrying. If incorrectly performed, these all add further stress to an already depleted support system. Chapters 2, 3 and 8 give further guidance. Guidelines for safe practice can be found in the Appendix.

SUMMARY

- Form and force closure of the pelvis are affected by pregnancy.
- PGP occurs in one in five pregnant women.
- Relaxin increases the elasticity of the collagen component of connective tissue.
- Joints continue to be at risk from the lingering effects of relaxin.
- Breastfeeding may prolong joint laxity.
- Posture must be retrained following

pregnancy, and essential back care learned during everyday baby care.

- Neutral spinal alignment should be adopted wherever possible.
- Postural adaptations should be considered in relation to exercise choice.
- All movements should be performed within the normal range of the joint.
- Overextension of any joint should be avoided.
- Correct joint alignment and exercise technique is vital.
- Flexibility work should be avoided until 16–20 weeks after delivery – longer if breast-feeding.
- High-impact activities should be avoided for the first few months after delivery.
- Reduced lumbopelvic stability affects all activities and increases the risk of injury.
- Recruitment of the deep stabilisers should be learned before adding resistance.
- Resistance programmes should be endurance-based.

REFERENCES

ACPWH (Association of Chartered Physiotherapists in Women's Health) 2007. Pregnancy-related pelvic girdle pain: Guidance for Health Professionals. Leaflet, ACPWH

Bani, D. 1997. Relaxin: A pleiotropic hormone. *General Pharmacology* 28(1): 13–22

Calleja-Agius, J. & Brincat, M.P. 2009. Effects of hormone replacement therapy on connective tissue: Why is this important? *Best Practice & Research: Clinical Obstetrics and Gynaecology* 23(1): 121–127

Foti, T., Davids, J.R. & Bagley, A. 2000. A biomechanical analysis of gait during pregnancy. *Journal of Bone Joint Surgery America* 82: 625–632

Gutke, A., Ostgaard, H.C. & Oberg, B. 2006. Pelvic girdle pain and lumbar pain in pregnancy: A cohort study of the consequences in terms of health and functioning. *Spine* 31: 149–55

Jain, N. & Sternberg, L.B. 2005. Symphyseal separation. *Obstetrics and Gynecology* 105: 1229–1232

Lee, D. 2007. *The Pelvic Girdle.* Oxford, Churchill Livingstone, (i) 45, (ii) 46 (iii) 101

Marnoch, M., Ramin, K., Ramsey, P., Song, S.W., Stensland, J.J. & An, K.N. 2003. Characterisation of the relationship between joint laxity and maternal hormones in pregnancy. *Obstetrics and Gynecology* 101(2): 331–335

Mercer, S. 2009. Anatomical and biomechanical evidence for the role of pelvic floor muscles as core stabilisers. Notes from presentation attended at the Conference of the International Organisation of Physical Therapists in Women's Health, Lisbon

O'Dwyer, M. 2009. Hold it sister – The confident physio's guide to core and floor rehabilitation. Seminar notes from presentation attended at St Thomas' Hospital, London

Richardson, C. 2008. www.gravityfit.com

Walsh, P. (Chair of the Association of Chartered Physiotherapists in Women's Health) 2008. Personal communication

LUMBOPELVIC STABILITY

2

As a child, you might have had a toy called a 'Weeble'. It was egg-shaped with a weighted base and you could push it in any direction without knocking it over – 'Weebles wobble but they don't fall down'. Weebles had a great stabilising system that allowed movement but maintained control.

Consider standing on a moving train with nothing to hold on to; instinctively the body will brace to resist the multi-directional movements, yet by allowing the body to roll with the flow, without stumbling or falling, the body can achieve stability with movement – just like a Weeble!

All too often, exercises are taught that encourage gripping, holding and bracing. While this may be necessary to support a heavy load, a high state of contraction interrupts the flow of the body and creates tension.

This chapter is about stability and mobility without rigidity and is appropriate for all clients, not just those who are postnatal!

What is stability?

Stability has nothing to do with strength – it relates to the effective functioning of a group of systems to control the body during movement.

The spinal stability system consists of three inter-relating subsystems (Panjabi 1992):

- **Passive system:** Joints/ligaments provide passive support
- **Active system:** Muscles provide active support
- **Control system**: Nerves co-ordinate sensory feedback from the other two systems

All systems should work together at the same level and they rely on each other to maintain equilibrium. However, in reality, one frequently works less than the others and compensatory changes will occur in the others. This can lead to musculoskeletal or neuromuscular problems.

Figure 2.1 Panjabi's model of the spinal stability system (1992)

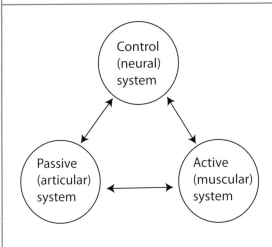

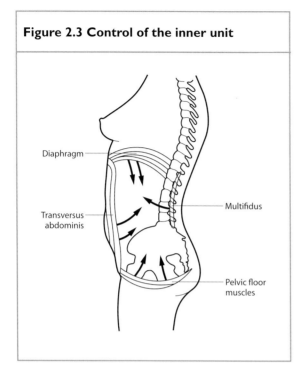

Figure 2.3 Control of the inner unit

Diaphragm

Transversus abdominis

Multifidus

Pelvic floor muscles

co-ordination with the diaphragm and TrA, and contract to resist intra-abdominal pressure (IAP) from above. O'Dwyer (2009) suggests the PFM are the key players in lumbopelvic stability, with problems occurring if they are either too weak or too strong.

How do the local stabilising muscles work?

Required to function at low intensities, these muscles are predominantly slow-twitch (Type I) and therefore do not need to be strong. A study by Cholewicki & McGill (1996) suggested that just a 1–3 per cent increase in muscle tension was sufficient to provide support. Recruitment is an automatic response by the central nervous system in anticipation of movement, load and displacement. In short they *respond* to movement but are not *responsible* for it – that is the job of the global muscles.

Low loads are associated with low levels of IAP and relaxed respiration (O'Sullivan 2005). If the load is predictable, as in a regular, low-level movement, the local system can manage on its own. If more support is required, or the load is unpredictable, the global muscles will assist. Support will always fluctuate between the two. Once movement is introduced, the global stabilisers must be helping (Comerford 2008). To optimise stability, muscles must work together in a sequential pattern, i.e. the local stabilisers activate first, followed by the global stabilisers.

How does this provide lumbopelvic stability?

Activation of TrA and multifidus tenses the thoracolumbar fascia, increasing joint stiffness. PFM activity increases on exhalation (Sapsford 2008) which means that as the diaphragm relaxes, the PFM contract. The combined effects increase IAP. When the local system is functioning optimally it provides anticipatory intersegmental control of the joints of the lumbar spine and pelvis (Hodges et al. 2003).

Stability is a continuum

In low-level movements when minimal effort is required to maintain joint control, the local

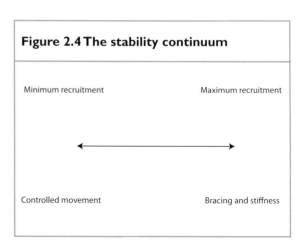

Figure 2.4 The stability continuum

Minimum recruitment   Maximum recruitment

Controlled movement   Bracing and stiffness

muscles can cope on their own. As limb movement increases, the local muscles need assistance from the global stabilisers to maintain alignment. At the higher-level end of the continuum, when maximum stability is needed, the local and global stabilisers together cannot cope so additional help is provided by the global mobilisers. Recruitment of the global mobilisers causes stability through bracing and stiffness.

Optimal recruitment patterns

Regardless of the load, all movements should begin with activation of the local stabilisers. The global muscles are then recruited to assist as required and activation fluctuates depending on the load. This is the optimal recruitment pattern for lumbopelvic stability.

CONTROL (NEURAL) SYSTEM

The neural system co-ordinates sensory feedback from the passive and active systems and is the vital link between the two. Proprioceptors are sensory nerve endings present in muscles, tendons, joint capsules and deep fascia and they provide information relating to body position and direction of movement. This information is relayed to the active system via the neural system so muscles can respond to make the necessary changes. The speed and accuracy of this messaging is crucial to the outcome.

Compensatory muscle patterning occurs as a result of injury, the threat of pain or postural change. The neuromuscular pathways are reorganised, altering proprioception, inhibiting motor neurons to drive muscles and heightening sensitivity to pain.

EFFECTS OF PREGNANCY AND DELIVERY ON THE STABILITY SYSTEMS

Table 2.1 shows how the passive, active and neural systems are affected by pregnancy and delivery. Reduced support from the passive system requires greater input from the active system, which is also undergoing change. This has compensatory effects on the neural system.

CURRENT RESEARCH

Most of the published research on lumbopelvic stabilisation has looked at patients with low back pain. These studies have all identified a dysfunction in the local muscle system, not relating to strength, but due to a timing deficit: these muscles switch on *after* loading (Hodges & Richardson 1996, Lee 2006). Hodges & Richardson (1996) suggest this timing delay is independent of the type or nature of pathology, i.e. disc, joint or nerve.

No studies to date have looked specifically at the effects of pregnancy and delivery on lumbopelvic stability. After consideration of the pregnancy changes outlined above, it has been assumed that a similar dysfunction may occur.

NON-OPTIMAL RECRUITMENT PATTERNS

Stability through rigidity

In the absence of effective support from the local system, the global stabilisers are activated to provide essential lumbopelvic support. Global mobilisers (e.g. hamstrings/erector spinae/iliopsoas) may be recruited to assist as required. While this is a natural strategy aimed at

Table 2.1	How the systems are affected by pregnancy and delivery
System	Effects
Passive	• Relaxin targets sites in pelvis to increase pelvic outlet • Increased weight and pressure from growing baby • Increased ligament laxity and reduced stability of lumbopelvic region • Lax connective tissue unable to transmit tension through fascia (as in diastasis recti) • Altered fascial tension in pelvic floor from organ displacement
Active	*Local muscles* • TrA and PFM lengthen under the strain • Atrophy due to unloading/mechanical weakness • Loss of co-ordination with other local muscles • Asymmetry due to lie of baby • Pelvic floor muscle and nerve damage *Global muscles* • Stabilisers lengthen and weaken (EO, gluteus maximus/medius) • Mobilisers shorten to take up the slack (piriformis, adductors, hamstrings) • Dominance of one or more mobilising muscles (erector spinae, iliopsoas) • Non-recruitment or asymmetrical activation of other muscles (gluteus maximus/medius) • Stretch-weakened RA and replacement with non-contractile tissue • Change in postural alignment
Control	• Loss of co-ordination with other local muscles • Altered recruitment patterning from pain and injury • Reduced sensory feedback • Timing delay in TrA/PFM/multifidus activation • Delayed offset of global stabilisers – stays switched on for longer (EO)

protecting the body from high loads, it is for intermittent use only. These larger muscles are designed for dynamic movement and not intended to work for prolonged periods of time. Working at higher frequencies than the local muscles, their recruitment will increase stiffness and achieve stability through rigidity.

If this system becomes the principal method of stabilisation, the mobilisers will shorten and tighten as they grip to hold on. Short, tight muscles pull the body out of alignment and create imbalance (*see* chapter 1). Poor postural alignment switches off the stabilising muscles (O'Dwyer 2009). Mis-recruitment compromises other functions, in particular balance, breathing and continence (Lee 2009).

Figure 2.4 Rib gripping

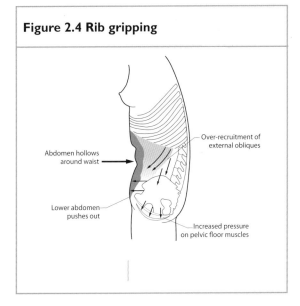

Abdomen hollows around waist →

Over-recruitment of external obliques

Lower abdomen pushes out

Increased pressure on pelvic floor muscles

Gripping evidence!

'Neurons that fire together, wire together' (Lee 2009). Having learned to over-recruit, these muscles will continue to fire up together until the wiring is fixed! Common sites for gripping are ribs, buttocks, and back. Postnatal women may fall into one, or all of these categories!

Gripping causes stiffness, and stiffness reduces movement. Movement is vital for the dissipation of forces so, unless the cycle is broken, muscular tension will continue to stress the structures and further problems may develop.

Rib grippers

Over-recruitment of the obliques is observed by the narrowing or hollowing of the abdomen around the waist and chest wall. Constant and sustained tightening of the abdomen (practised by many women, not just postnatal mums) will create this appearance. This restricts rotation and extension of the trunk and causes disordered breathing. Learning to breathe correctly is essential for rib grippers (*see* page 20). O'Dwyer (2009) suggests that rigidity causes hypertrophy of IO/EO, increasing the risk of prolapse (*see* chapter 4).

Buttock grippers

Over-recruitment of the deep lateral rotators of the hip (particularly piriformis) to aid pelvic stability can be observed by creases in the clothing around the buttock line and an indentation felt in the shape of the buttocks around the side (Lee 2007). This forces the head of the femur into the front of the acetabulum, and changes to the pattern of gait may lead to hip

Figure 2.5 Buttock gripping

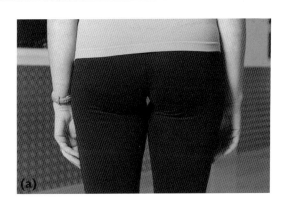
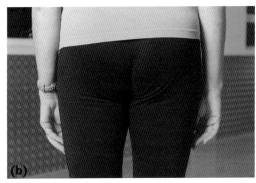

(a)

(b)

or groin pain. Buttock grippers can also be identified by poor squatting technique as they will be unable to flex comfortably at the hips: the buttocks will tuck under and the back will round forwards. Seated posture will also display a posterior pelvic tilt. Releasing the buttocks and learning to take the trunk forwards during squatting is recommended.

Back grippers

Increased stiffness of the spinal extensors, long weak RA, and anterior tilt or forward sway of the pelvis are the perfect recipe for a back gripper. This action causes stiffness and discomfort in the mid or low back, especially during prolonged standing. Back grippers can be identified during squatting when the lumbar and cervical spines both hyperextend. Focus should be on maintaining the same distance between the breast bone and the pubic bone (i.e. maintaining neutral pelvis) during squatting. Stretching the back muscles is also recommended.

TRAINING RECOMMENDATIONS

- Adopt correct postural alignment.
- Learn to breathe correctly.
- Train the brain to recruit the deep stabilisers prior to movement.

Postural alignment

Adopting an upright posture in sitting and standing switches on the inner unit. Slumping or slouching shuts down TrA and the PFM and prevents the diaphragm from moving down during inhalation (O'Dwyer 2009). Encouraging a lengthened spine with correct alignment turns on the deep stabilisers and is the No. 1 exercise for local muscle endurance!

Breathing techniques

Poor breathing patterns restrict the movement of the diaphragm and this will affect inner unit activation. Upper chest breathing prevents the diaphragm from moving freely: the ribs are 'fixed' and breathing becomes shallow, increasing tension in the neck and shoulders as the accessory breathing muscles overwork. A tight bra or belt has the same effect! O'Dwyer (2009) suggests this breathing pattern is common in busy, high-achieving women who are always on the go, don't stop and relax and are unable to 'let go'. This could include some of our clients – maybe ourselves too!

Many emotions are 'held' in the abdomen and pulling in the waist is part of our female psyche. If this 'holding' is done by RA/EO, the diaphragm, the PFM and TrA cannot function properly. Lee (2007) confirms it is essential to teach correct diaphragmatic breathing to restore lumbopelvic function. While this may seem a rather basic, time-consuming practice, it is an essential first stage of lumbopelvic stability training, which should not progress until women are competent.

Teaching correct breathing patterns

- Position hands on lower ribcage with fingers facing inwards.
- Inhale, taking the breath into the lower ribcage and abdomen, keeping RA/EO relaxed.
- Feel the ribs opening sideways and the abdomen swelling.
- As you exhale, *relax* the ribcage and feel the diaphragm lifting up.

Relaxing the abdomen on exhalation and letting it soften and swell may be very difficult for some women. After years of holding in, it may take time to feel comfortable with letting go. Encouragement, empathy and praise are required. Practise when side/supine lying, seated and standing and keep checking for substitution.

Once the local stabilisers can be correctly recruited in a co-ordinated way, breathing cues should be avoided. Stipulating specific breathing patterns will compromise respiration, increase thoracic tension and encourage rib gripping. Breath holding should be avoided at all times. Breathing exercises are recommended during quiet times.

Diaphragmatic breathing has additional benefits for postnatal women by increasing thoracic mobility. Pregnancy-induced changes to the musculoskeletal and respiratory systems increase sternum and ribcage stiffness and reduce movement in the thoracic spine. During inhalation the breath should be directed into the lower part of the lungs so that the lower ribcage moves sideways and backwards to massage and loosen the thoracic spine. A long exhalation promotes a more relaxed state and should be encouraged. Diaphragmatic breathing stimulates the parasympathetic nervous system that calms the body and slows down the breathing rate; the 'rest and digest' response is far more appropriate than the 'fight or flight' response of the sympathetic nervous system.

Train the brain

The brain doesn't differentiate between muscles so when learning a new movement it recruits what it thinks it needs to do the job. Unfamiliar movements feel awkward and uncoordinated but become more refined with practice. Recruitment reduces as the body becomes more skilled: the brain responds faster and relegates the activity to the background. Once the brain can pre-empt the movement it becomes a learned response. An incorrect movement pattern can be learned this way too.

Lee (2009) believes you can't strengthen a muscle that your brain isn't using! This is partic-ularly relevant to programmes claiming to be for 'core strengthening' – unless the brain is able to recruit the deep stabilising muscles, such activities may just be reinforcing a faulty muscle recruitment pattern.

Non-optimal movement patterns must be undone and the brain retrained to recruit correctly. Hodges (2009) suggests it is not enough to simply activate the muscle: it must be skill-related. So to change motor control the brain–muscle connection must be trained in functional positions, as the information is not transferable! (*See* page 29, Multi-positional training for TrA.)

Retrain correct muscle recruitment

- Encourage upright posture to train the inner unit.
- Pre-activate TrA before each exercise commences.
- Once fired up, TrA will continue to work *for the duration of that movement pattern.*
- Reminders are *unnecessary and inappropriate.*
- Re-activate before starting a new exercise.
- Relax the muscles that are gripping – work less and learn to switch off.
- Use functional positions.

If it's not broken, don't try to fix it!

If local stabilisers are activated without conscious control they will not need reminders to switch on: once the movement pattern has been correctly learned, stop talking about it! Continued cueing will result in overactivity and rigidity.

Balance movement with stability

Postnatal women need to breathe correctly, free up tensions in the thoracic spine and relax the muscles that are gripping. Once the local muscles have regained their role in lumbopelvic stability the body can move freely again. This is the aim for retraining postnatal women.

Exercises to improve lumbopelvic stability can be found in chapter 3.

SUMMARY

- Stability has nothing to do with strength.
- It involves three interrelated systems: active, passive and control.
- Systems must work together to be effective.
- Local stabilising muscles are diaphragm, multifidus, TrA and the PFM.
- Local stabilisers are located deep inside the trunk and together they form a cylinder of stability.
- Recruited at low frequencies, they are continuously active.
- Global stabilising muscles are recruited at higher intensities and work for short periods at a time.
- Global stabilisers assist local muscles when demand increases.
- Pregnancy and birth disrupt the effectiveness of local stabilisers.
- Dysfunction in local muscles requires input from global stabilisers.
- Muscles not designed to work for long periods will shorten and tighten.
- Short, tight muscles pull the body out of alignment.
- Over-recruitment causes fatigue.
- Brain needs to be trained to recruit local stabilising muscles prior to movement.
- Postural alignment and correct breathing is essential.

REFERENCES

Cholewicki, J. & McGill, S. 1996. Mechanical stability in the lumbar spine: implications for injury and chronic low back pain. *Clinical Biomechanics* 11(1): 1–15

Comerford, M.J. 2008. The truth about transversus: Clinical application of the research. Seminar notes from presentation attended at University College London

Comerford, M.J. & Mottram, S.L. 2001. Movement and stability dysfunction – contemporary developments. *Manual Therapy* 6(1): 15–26

Cresswell, A.G. & Thorstensson, A. 1994. Changes in intra-abdominal pressure, trunk muscle activation and force during isokinetic lifting and lowering. *European Journal of Applied Occupational Physiology* 68: 315–21

Hodges, P.W. 1999. Is there a role for transversus abdominis in lumbo-pelvic stability? *Manual Therapy* 4(2): 74–86

Hodges, P.W. 2009. Moving on from giving isolated core stability exercises. Seminar notes from presentation attended at University College London

Hodges, P.W., Holm, A.K., Holm, T.S., Elkstrom, T.L., Cresswell, A., Hansson, T. & Thorstensson, A. 2003. Intervertebral stiffness of the spine is increased by evoked contraction of transversus abdominis and the diaphragm: In vivo porcine studies. *Spine* 28: 2594–601

Hodges, P.W. & Richardson C.A. 1996. Inefficient muscular stabilization of the lumbar spine associated with low back pain: A motor control evaluation of transverses abdominis. *Spine* 21: 2640

Lee, D. 2007. *The Pelvic Girdle*. Oxford: Churchill Livingstone, 192

Lee, L.J. 2006. Is it possible to be too stable? *Orthopaedic Division Review* Nov/Dec

Lee, L.J. 2009. Moving on from giving isolated

core stability exercises. Seminar notes from presentation attended at University College London

MacDonald, D.A., Moseley, G.L. and Hodges, P.W. 2006. The lumbar multifidus: Does the evidence support clinical beliefs? *Manual Therapy* 11(4): 254–263

Myers, T. 2000. Cups and domes. *Massage therapy* Aug/Sep (*see* also www.massagetherapy.com/articles)

O'Dwyer, M. 2009. Hold it sister – The confident physio's guide to core and floor rehabilitation. Seminar notes from presentation attended at St Thomas' Hospital, London

O'Sullivan, P. 2005. Diagnosis and classification of chronic low back pain disorders: Maladaptive movement and motor control impairments as underlying mechanism. *Manual Therapy* 10(4): 242–55

Panjabi, M.M. 1992. The stabilising system of the spine. Part I: Function, dysfunction, adaptation and enhancement. *Journal of Spinal Disorders* 5(4): 383–9

Sapsford, R.R. 2008. Co-ordination of the abdominal and pelvic floor muscles. PhD Thesis, University of Queensland

THE ABDOMINAL MUSCLES

3

STRUCTURE OF THE ABDOMINAL MUSCLES

The four abdominal muscles – transversus abdominis, internal oblique, external oblique and rectus abdominis – interconnect to form a muscular corset. They are very closely linked through connective tissue and rarely work alone.

Transversus abdominis

Transversus abdominis (TrA) is the deepest of the four muscles (*see* fig. 3.1a). Arising from the

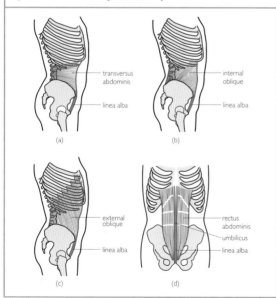

Figure 3.1 The four abdominal muscles: a) transversus abdominis, b) internal oblique, c) external oblique and d) rectus abdominis

thoracolumbar fascia, lower six ribs, iliac crest and the inguinal ligament, the muscle wraps horizontally around the torso and the two sides insert into a broad tendinous band at the front called the abdominal aponeurosis. The lower fibres curve downwards and attach on to the pubis. The aponeurosis of TrA joins with the aponeurosis of the obliques at the midline of the body to form the linea alba. TrA is believed to play a significant role in stabilising the linea alba (Sheppard 1996, Boissonnault & Kotarinos 1988).

The linea alba is a tendinous raphe, seen along the midline of the abdomen between the inner borders of rectus abdominis. It is formed by the blending of the aponeuroses from both sides of the TrA and obliques. It is narrower below than above the umbilicus, corresponding with the width of rectus abdominis as it ascends.

Together with the internal oblique, TrA supports the abdominal organs and in association with the other local stabilisers, namely multifidus, pelvic floor muscles and diaphragm, provides lumbopelvic stability. Many studies indicate that the role of TrA is to activate prior to movement to increase stiffness and stability of the spine (Cresswell 1993, Hodges & Richardson 1996). It is the only muscle to be active in all trunk movements in all directions and its activity always precedes that of the other abdominal muscles in normal subjects (Norris 2000). TrA is also a muscle of respiration (Comerford 2008) and interdigitates with the diaphragm in its attachments onto the ribs. See chapter 2 for further discussion.

Internal oblique

The internal oblique (IO) lies on top of the TrA muscle and forms an inverted V shape (*see* fig. 3.1b). Like TrA, its origins are thoracolumbar fascia, iliac crest and inguinal ligament, and its fibres run inwards to the linea alba, upwards to the lower four ribs and downwards to the pubis. As with TrA this muscle feeds into its own aponeurosis which forms part of the linea alba, as described above. The aponeurosis of the IO is particularly significant as it subdivides at the outer edges of rectus abdominis and passes in front of and behind the rectus muscle, encasing it within an aponeurotic sheath, before rejoining at the linea alba. This occurs on the upper two-thirds of rectus abdominis only; in the lower third (just below the umbilicus) the three layers of aponeuroses of the TrA, IO and external oblique pass over the top of rectus abdominis. Due to the variable direction of their fibres, IO can assist TrA with abdominal compression, flex the trunk to the same side and work with external oblique on the opposite side to rotate the trunk.

External oblique

The external oblique (EO) lies on top of, and perpendicular to, the IO and forms an upright V shape (*see* fig. 3.1c). It originates on the lower eight ribs and runs diagonally and vertically downwards to insert onto the iliac crest. The midline attachment feeds into its own aponeurosis which passes over the top of rectus abdominis and meets with its opposite number in the centre to form the linea alba. It interdigitates with serratus anterior at the top and latissimus dorsi below. EO works together with IO from the opposite side to rotate the trunk. It also assists rectus abdominis with trunk flexion.

Rectus abdominis

Rectus abdominis (RA) forms the central structure of the abdominal muscles. It is made up of two bands of muscle that begin on the pubic bone, and travel upwards to attach onto the sternum and 5th, 6th, 7th ribs (*see* fig. 3.1d). It is narrower at the bottom and increases in width to approximately 15cm at the top. The muscle has three fibrous bands, known as tendinous inscriptions, or intersections, that pass transversely across in a zigzag course: one at the level of the umbilicus, one at the xiphoid process (base of the sternum) and the third midway between the two. Sometimes one or two additional inscriptions, generally incomplete, are present below the umbilicus. These fibrous bands are believed to be a safety feature as RA is a very long muscle passing over an empty space. Separating them into four smaller muscles, rather than one long strip, reduces the risk of tearing if overstretched (Myers 1998).

The position of the lowest inscription is particularly relevant when checking for separation of the muscles (*see* page 44) as the area around the umbilicus is the weakest. Each side of RA is encased in a sheath made from the aponeuroses of the oblique and TrA muscles. These merge together in the centre to form the linea alba. In the lower third of the abdomen, the aponeuroses pass over the top of the RA, making the muscle less visible.

Pyramidalis

Discussion of the abdominal group would not be complete without mention of this tiny pyramid-shaped muscle, made of two halves, situated in the rectus sheath in front of the RA bands. Pyramidalis begins on the pubis and inserts into the lower portion of the linea alba – between the umbilicus and the pubis. Its precise function is unclear but together the two sides are thought to tense the linea alba.

It is absent in approximately 20 per cent of the population (Lovering & Anderson 2007) and may occur on one side only. It has been suggested that its absence may increase the risk of diastasis recti but no studies to date have explored this.

FUNCTIONS OF THE ABDOMINAL MUSCLES

The abdominal muscles:
- stabilise and support the pelvis and lumbar spine;
- support the abdominal and pelvic organs;
- flex the trunk to one side;
- curl the trunk forwards;
- rotate the trunk;
- maintain correct pelvic alignment;
- increase IAP, i.e. during coughing or sneezing, lifting;
- aid expulsive movements, e.g. vomiting, excretion and during the second stage of labour;
- assist expiration.

PREGNANCY AND THE ABDOMINAL MUSCLES

What happens to the abdominal muscles during pregnancy?

Under the influence of relaxin the abdominal muscles undergo a tremendous amount of stretching, in all directions, to accommodate the growing baby. Connective tissue within and around the muscles provides a degree of elasticity, but the main changes occur in the linea alba. Relaxin increases the elasticity of the collagen component of connective tissue and this allows the linea alba to stretch in both directions. The waistline may increase by approximately 50cm and RA lengthen by approximately 20cm. Recent studies suggest that RA may also widen and thin as it is stretched in both directions (Coldron et al. 2007).

The two bands of muscle which previously lay parallel stretch away from the midline to allow more space for the growing uterus. This is known as 'diastasis recti' – separation of the recti muscles. It is a normal structural adaptation occurring in 66 per cent of women in the third trimester, 27 per cent separating earlier, in the second trimester (Boissonnault & Blaschak 1988). The majority of women will be unaware of this change, although it is not uncommon to experience backache due to the reduced support from the abdominal muscles. Very little research has been done into the effects of pregnancy on the other three abdominal muscles – the majority of research currently available relates to the changes occurring in RA.

Stretch weakness

Stretch weakness occurs when a muscle remains elongated, beyond its normal resting position, but not beyond the normal range of muscle length (Kendall et al. 1993). In this position, its contractile ability is reduced, as the actin and

Figure 3.2 Abdominal muscles during pregnancy

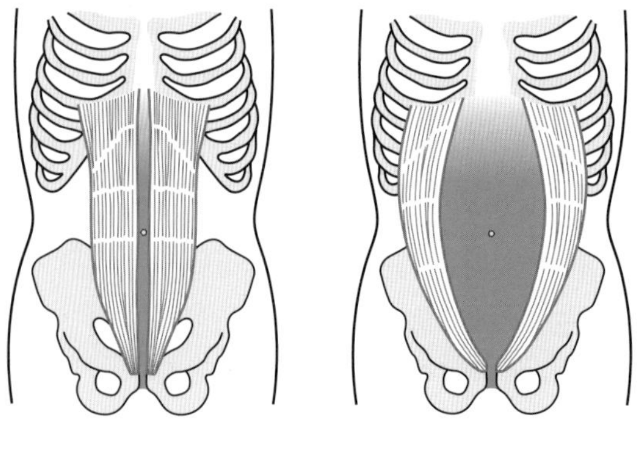

myosin filaments have been taken too far apart. The muscle adapts by adding another sarcomere to the end of the muscle fibre, which pushes the contractile elements closer together. This adaptation can occur in any muscle as a result of prolonged stretch but is particularly relevant to RA as it stretches over the pregnant uterus.

Stretch-weakened muscles have a reduced ability to maintain full contraction in the inner range (Norris 2000) and this may be related to a change in muscle fibre type. Animal studies indicate an alteration in muscle fibre type as a result of prolonged stretch and Coldron et al. (2007) suggest this may occur in RA during the latter half of pregnancy, with an increase in Type I fibres and a decrease in Type IIA. This would explain the apparent loss of strength in inner range.

Muscle length usually reduces following birth but it should not be assumed that this has occurred. The process can be speeded up by exercises to shorten RA and inner-range training.

What happens during a caesarean section?

Trauma to the abdominal muscles during a caesarean section is not as severe as many women believe, as the muscles themselves are not cut. An incision of approximately 10cm is made into the skin, just above the pubic bone to expose the rectus sheath, which is also cut. In this part of the abdomen the rectus sheath (aponeuroses) passes over the top of RA; therefore, once the sheath has been cut, the two sides of RA can be drawn apart. Further incisions are made into the peritoneum (lining of the abdominal cavity) and the uterus before the baby is lifted. Repair involves stitching the uterus, peritoneum and the skin; the RA muscles are drawn back together and the rectus sheath is realigned.

Is it more difficult for the muscles to recover after a caesarean?

Most women who deliver by caesarean section feel that abdominal recovery is inhibited by the procedure. Although the muscles have not been cut, the layers of aponeuroses have, and there has been a certain amount of abdominal disruption, leaving bruising and bloating. It is for this reason that women may have more difficulty recruiting TrA. Trapped air may add to the problem in the first couple of days post-delivery. This can be relieved by performing pelvic tilts in a supine position. Tingling and numbness will be experienced around the scar site, with sensation returning in patches; full sensory recovery could take up to six months.

Abdominal muscle recovery

Three to four days after the baby is born, RA will begin to realign and the wide separation gradually reduces. By eight weeks in most cases it will have recovered to approximately two finger widths (20mm) apart at the umbilicus, and many women will find that recovery plateaus at this point (Coldron et al. 2007). Several layers of stretched tissue remain and most women will feel a lack of support in the abdomen. Gentle exercises to encourage RA to shorten and come together will be invaluable in the early postnatal period and will speed up recovery time. These exercises are usually advised on discharge from hospital but are frequently misunderstood or not performed! Training correct recruitment of TrA is essential. See chapter 6 for discussion on persistent diastasis recti.

Implications for muscle strength

In addition to the alteration in muscle fibre types from Type I to IIA, other changes occur to the structure and composition of RA that may contribute to decreased strength. Studies by Coldron et al. (2007) suggest that the thickness of RA is reduced during pregnancy and some of the contractile components may be replaced by fat and connective tissue. Stelzner et al. (1993) suggest that stretch-induced denervation of the abdominal wall may occur during pregnancy and delivery and this will reduce muscle activation. Considering all these factors it is not surprising that women experience a decrease in abdominal muscle strength!

Care of the abdominal muscles

The abdominal muscles may remain stretched and weakened for some time, prolonging their vulnerability and reducing spinal support. Guidance on correct performance of everyday tasks is essential and should be included in every postnatal programme. See Appendix.

What are the aims of postnatal abdominal muscle re-training?

- Re-educate recruitment of TrA in all functional movements to improve lumbopelvic stability
- Shorten RA and realign the muscle bellies
- Strengthen RA within its inner range
- Strengthen the rest of the abdominal group to improve functional fitness

How soon should abdominal exercises commence?

Abdominal training should begin as soon as possible after delivery – ideally within 24 hours. Level 1 TrA and pelvic tilting in all positions are suitable to do in the first few days after delivery and these are often given out by the hospital on discharge. Gentle recruitment of TrA should be encouraged throughout the day in association with dynamic tasks: getting out of bed, standing up, bending down etc.

RE-EDUCATION OF TrA

Why is this a priority?

TrA is a deep postural muscle that, together with other local stabilisers, is responsible for maintaining lumbopelvic stability. It doesn't need to be strong but it needs to activate prior to movement to provide support. Changes to the abdominal musculature during pregnancy seem to alter the recruitment pattern of the deep stabilisers, necessitating the activation of other muscles to help out. Mis-recruitment compromises other functions, in particular balance, breathing and continence (Hodges & Lee 2009). Relearning correct activation is an important first step, so it is important to dedicate sufficient time and emphasis to re-education before progressing. This is discussed in more detail in chapter 4.

Locating and activating TrA

- Standing or sitting in an upright position, place your fingers on your hip bones at the front of the pelvis (ASIS).
- Move your fingers diagonally downwards and inwards approximately 2.5cm into the soft tissue of the abdomen – you should be directly on top of TrA and IO.
- Apply gentle pressure into the soft tissue and cough several times.
- As you cough you should feel TrA and IO contract as they resist the rise in IAP.
- Now try to create the same feeling, without coughing, by drawing your abdomen in very softly.
- It may help to imagine a wire between the two ASIS, gently drawing them together.
- Feel the muscles working underneath your fingers.
- This is all that is required to fire up TrA – nothing more!

Encourage minimal recruitment in all positions (i.e. side and supine lying, sitting, standing, kneeling etc.) and emphasise the importance of activating prior to movement. Recommend practice with everyday baby care, particularly when lifting or carrying. This trains the brain to pre-activate in this way, to provide a stable base for larger movements. Research suggests that TrA works most effectively in neutral spine (Sapsford et al. 2001), so adoption of this alignment is recommended wherever possible. This is explained in the exercise section of this chapter.

Once fired up, TrA should continue to work for the duration of that movement pattern. Constant reminders to draw in the abdomen will encourage recruitment of other muscles and defeat the object. Instructors are advised to review their teaching habits to ensure that this doesn't happen.

Problems contracting TrA

Although it appears incredibly simple, this movement takes time to learn and perform correctly – true of a great percentage of people, not just postnatal women. Common errors include breath holding, buttock squeezing and bracing the abdomen. To contract effectively and create sufficient stability for the spine, TrA only needs to work at 25 per cent of its maximum (Richardson et al. 1995). A soft sinking feeling, rather like a balloon deflating in the abdomen, is all that is required, but many women will brace and pull in strongly while inhaling. This action recruits RA and EO and overrides the action of TrA. Look out for a strong depression in the ribcage, accompanied by a horizontal crease across the upper abdomen, as this will indicate these muscles are being incorrectly recruited. Postnatal women are particularly at risk with this action as it increases pressure on the pelvic floor, with major consequences for the stability of the pelvic organs (O'Dwyer 2009) (*see* chapter 4).

TrA and pelvic floor co-ordination

As two key players in the inner unit, TrA and the PFM work together to provide lumbopelvic stability. Studies by Sapsford (2008) suggest that voluntary activation of the abdominal or pelvic floor muscles in healthy women influences activity in the other muscle group. Results of these studies varied depending on the position of the lumbar spine, with reduced activation in slumped postures.

However, postnatal women with stretched, weakened abdominal muscles and dysfunctional PFM may not experience such co-ordination so it cannot be assumed that co-activation will occur. Studies by Hodges & Richardson (1996) and Lee (2006) suggest that poor inner unit co-ordination is not associated with muscle strength but due to a change in recruitment patterning (*see* chapter 2).

Multi-positional training for TrA

When learning to recruit TrA correctly it is recommended to commence with floor-based exercises, as this provides useful feedback on the maintenance of correct alignment. Once correct activation has been learned it is important to train TrA to function in all positions, as activities of daily living are multi-positional. Adopting upright spinal alignment should be encouraged as often as possible and the avoidance of slumped positions, while both sitting and standing, should be stressed.

Finding neutral spine

Before commencing any exercise it is essential to position the body correctly to maximise the effectiveness of TrA.

The following instructions for finding correct body positioning should be used and reinforced before commencing an exercise. They are also useful as exercises in themselves. Instructions for correct standing alignment can be found on page 8.

Figure 3.3 Neutral spinal alignment in supine: a) Anterior tilt, b) Posterior tilt, c) Neutral

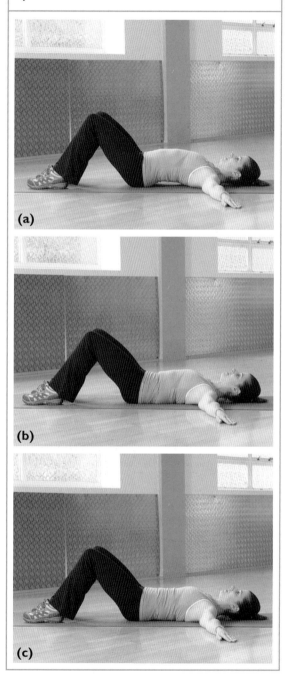

(a)

(b)

(c)

Supine

- Lie on your back with knees bent and feet flat on the floor, hip-width apart (hip-width should be taken from the position of ASIS (hip bones) and not the outside of the thighs).
- Place heel of hands on hip bones and fingertips on pubic bone.
- Gently roll the pelvis forwards (pubic bone downwards) so that your back arches off the floor, and the fingertips lower (anterior tilt).
- Gently roll the pelvis the opposite way so that your lower back presses into the floor and the fingertips lift (posterior tilt).
- Find a position midway between these two extremes where the lower back forms a natural curve and heel of hands/fingertips are on the same horizontal plane.
- This is your neutral pelvic position.

NB: This should only involve movement of the bones – there should be no muscular contraction involved in holding the position. Allow yourself a few seconds to relax into position, then go through the following checkpoints:

- Equal weight between right and left foot
- Shoulder blades sliding down your back
- Arms lengthening away from shoulders
- Breastbone relaxed
- Nose in line with breastbone and pubic bone
- Spine long

This is your neutral spine and will be referred to throughout the programme in the exercise preparation section.

Side lying

This position is frequently adopted incorrectly as it is often difficult for individuals to feel it for themselves – instructor observation is essential.

- Lie on your side with head resting on small cushion or on underneath arm.

- Rest the top arm on the floor for support.
- Bend the knees and stack the hips one on top of the other.
- Lift the waist to prevent pelvis tipping (a rolled up towel can be used as a prop if required).
- Find neutral pelvis using the anterior and posterior pelvic tilts as before, moving in a slow, controlled way.
- Keep back of head in line with mid-thoracic spine and sacrum.
- Lengthen the chest and open the top shoulder.
- Place a towel under the lower hip if required for comfort.

Four-point kneeling

This is another difficult one for individuals to feel for themselves – instructor observation is essential.

- Position knees under hips and hands under shoulders, fingers facing forwards.
- Distribute weight equally between knees and hands.
- Find neutral pelvis using the anterior and posterior pelvic tilts as before, moving in a slow, controlled way.

Figure 3.4 Neutral spinal alignment: a) arching the back, b) neutral spine, c) pressing the lower back into the floor

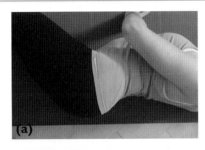
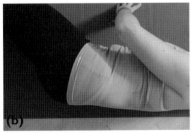
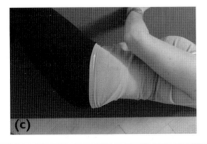

Figure 3.5 Neutral spinal alignment: a) anterior tilt, b) neutral spine, c) posterior tilt

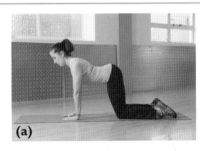
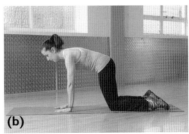
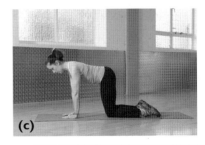

- Keep back of head in line with mid-thoracic spine and sacrum.
- Push gently away from the hands without flexing thoracic spine.
- Slide the shoulder blades down and soften the elbows.
- Lengthen the spine.

Seated

The following relates to any seated position – floor, chair or stability ball.

- Sit down, with knees bent and feet flat on the floor, hip-width apart.
- Lengthen the spine.
- Find neutral pelvis using the anterior and posterior pelvic tilts as before, moving in a slow, controlled way.
- Relax front of thighs.
- Feel your body weight supported by your sit bones.
- Slide shoulder blades down your back.
- Keep back of head in line with mid-thoracic spine and sacrum.

Figure 3.6 Neutral spinal alignment: a) anterior tilt, b) neutral spine, c) posterior tilt

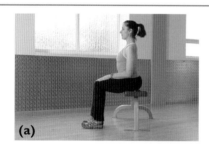

(a)

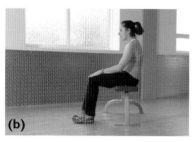

(b)

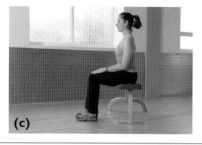

(c)

EXERCISES FOR TRAINING TrA RECRUITMENT TO IMPROVE LUMBOPELVIC STABILITY

Level 1

The following exercises are designed to recruit TrA and other local muscles to improve lumbopelvic stability during low-level movement of the limbs. They should be performed slowly and thoughtfully, utilising full range of movement to maximise benefits. Increasing speed and momentum at this stage may necessitate the activation of the mobilisers to provide stability, rendering the exercise ineffective for its purpose. The upper body exercises are particularly helpful for increasing thoracic mobility and assisting ribcage closure. The pattern of breathing should focus on exhaling with recruitment of TrA to ensure that the local stabilisers are working together as a group. These exercises should be cued for the first repetition and breathing encouraged throughout. It is not necessary to give constant reminders to activate TrA – once they have been recruited they should continue to work for the duration of the exercise.

Scissor arms

Preparation

Lie supine in neutral spinal alignment. Float the arms up towards the ceiling at chest height until directly above shoulders. Release the shoulder blades into the floor.

Action

Inhale to prepare and as you exhale recruit TrA and lower the right arm towards the floor above the head and the left arm down by your side. Keep the ribcage soft. Return the arms towards the ceiling at chest height and repeat, alternating the arms.

Technique tips

- Maintain neutral spine throughout.
- Range of movement is determined by the ability to keep the ribcage on the floor. This may be limited for some individuals – if the ribcage begins to lift, the arms have gone too far and stabilisation is lost.
- Think of moving the arms from the middle of the back rather than from the shoulders.
- Lengthen the arms away from the shoulders.

Figure 3.7 Scissor arms

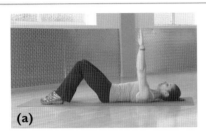
(a)

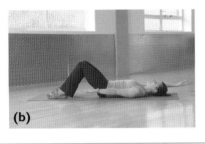
(b)

Figure 3.8 Chest flye

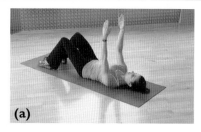

(a)

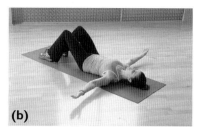

(b)

Chest flye

Preparation

Lie supine in neutral spinal alignment. Float the arms up towards the ceiling at chest height until directly above shoulders. Release the shoulder blades into the floor.

Action

Inhale to prepare and as you exhale recruit TrA and lower the arms to the side towards the floor at chest height. Keep the ribcage soft and draw the shoulder blades down as they open. Return the arms towards the ceiling and repeat.

Technique tips

- Maintain neutral spine throughout.
- Range of movement is determined by the ability to keep the ribcage on the floor. This may be limited for some individuals – if the ribcage begins to lift, the arms have gone too far and stabilisation is lost.
- Think of moving the arms from the middle of the back rather than from the shoulders.
- Lengthen the arms away from the shoulders.

Figure 3.9 Arm circle

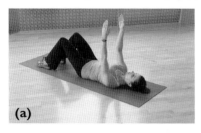

(a)

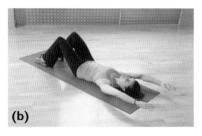

(b)

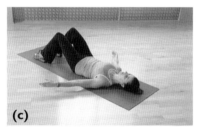

(c)

Arm circle

Preparation

Lie supine in neutral spinal alignment. Float the arms up towards the ceiling at chest height until directly above shoulders. Release the shoulder blades into the floor.

Action

Inhale to prepare and as you exhale recruit TrA and lower both arms towards the floor above the head, keeping the ribcage soft. Pause here before circling both arms around and down by your sides, scooping the air and drawing the shoulder blades down. Lift the arms back up to the ceiling and repeat.

Technique tips

- Maintain neutral spine throughout.
- Range of movement is determined by the ability to keep the ribcage on the floor. This may be limited for some individuals – if the ribcage begins to lift, the arms have gone too far and stabilisation is lost.
- Think of moving the arms from the middle of the back rather than from the shoulders.
- Lengthen the arms away from the shoulders.

Figure 3.10 Leg slide

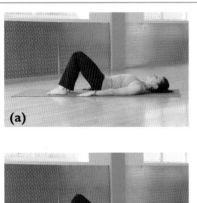

(a)

(b)

Leg slide

Preparation

Lie supine with neutral spinal alignment.

Action

Inhale to prepare and as you exhale recruit TrA and slowly slide one leg out along the floor until the knee straightens. Pause in the extended position to check that neutral alignment hasn't been lost. Slide the leg back up to the starting position and repeat, alternating the legs.

Technique tips

- Lengthen the leg away from the hip.
- Avoid rocking the pelvis.
- Avoid locking out the knee.
- Soften the ribcage into the floor.
- Keep the upper body stable throughout.

Progression

Perform with scissor arms using opposite arm to leg. Progress further using same arm as leg, maintaining neutral spine throughout.

Figure 3.11 Bent knee fall-out

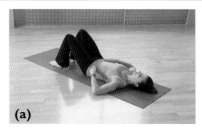

(a)

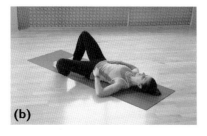

(b)

Bent knee fall-out

This exercise is useful for controlled lengthening of the adductors (*see* section on PGP in chapter 6) and can be done lying parallel to the wall to limit range of movement and encourage relaxation of the adductors.

Preparation

Lie supine in neutral spinal alignment. Bend elbows and rest fingertips on hip bones.

Action

Inhale to prepare and as you exhale recruit TrA and open the right knee to the side, allowing the foot to roll outwards but without lifting the opposite hip. Pause in the open position and check that neutral alignment hasn't been lost. Return the knee to starting position and repeat, alternating the legs.

Technique tips

- Keep the pelvis level throughout – check this with hands on hips.
- Range of movement is dependent on the maintenance of pelvic alignment.
- Do not allow the other knee to drop out to counterbalance the movement – keep it pointing up to the ceiling.
- Soften the ribcage into the floor as the leg moves away, to maintain spinal alignment.
- Keep the upper body relaxed throughout.
- Lengthen the arms away from the shoulders.
- Perform slowly and with control.

Caution: Stop immediately if any discomfort is felt in the SP or SIJ.

Figure 3.12 Knee raise

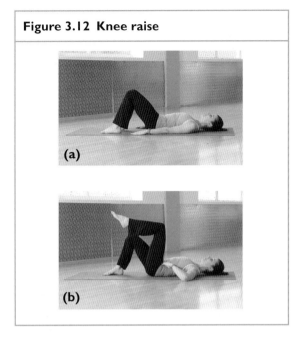

(a)

(b)

Knee raise

Preparation

Lie supine in neutral spinal alignment.

Action

Inhale to prepare and as you exhale recruit TrA and peel one foot slowly off the floor, bringing your knee up over the hip. Pause and check that neutral alignment hasn't been lost. Lower the leg slowly, maintaining neutral spine. Repeat, alternating the legs.

Technique tips

- Maintain neutral alignment throughout.
- Avoid sinking into the floor as the leg lifts, or arching as it lowers.
- Lift the foot slowly to encourage more effective work.
- Avoid pressing down on the supporting foot.
- Soften the ribcage and keep the upper body relaxed.
- Slide the shoulder blades down.

Figure 3.13 Kneeling leg and arm raise

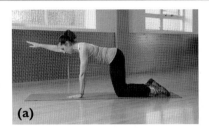

(a)

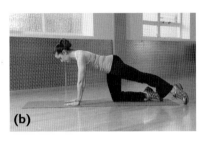

(b)

Kneeling leg and arm raise

Preparation

In four-point kneeling with spine in neutral alignment (*see* page 31).

Action

Perform the following as two separate movements:

1 Inhale to prepare and as you exhale recruit TrA and slide one arm forwards, lengthening from the fingertips as the arm lifts. Aim to lift it until parallel to the floor. Pause and check that neutral alignment hasn't been lost and slide the shoulder blades down. Lower and repeat on alternate sides.
2 Inhale to prepare and as you exhale recruit TrA and slide one foot out along the floor, keeping the pelvis level and lengthening the leg away from you. Pause and check that neutral alignment hasn't been lost, then slide the leg slowly back in again. Repeat on alternate sides.

Progression

• Combine the two movements, using opposite arm and leg.
• As above, but lift the leg off the floor.

Level 2

These exercises will require more assistance from the global stabilisers than in Level 1. As before, they should be performed slowly and thoughtfully, commencing with a small range of movement and increasing as stability improves. Speed and momentum will necessitate the activation of the larger mobilising muscles, rendering them ineffective for their purpose. Breathing and TrA cueing are as before.

Figure 3.14 Knee roll

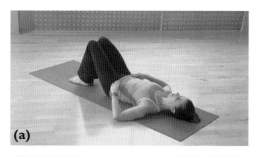

(a)

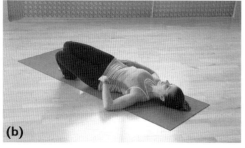

(b)

Knee roll

This exercise is particularly good for increasing spinal mobility but requires activation of the obliques.

Important!

Knee roll is not suitable for women with PEP nor for those with an RA separation of more than two fingers.

Preparation

Lie supine in neutral spinal alignment, but with feet together.

Action

Inhale to prepare and as you exhale recruit TrA and slowly lower the knees towards the floor to the left, allowing the right buttock to lift but keeping the ribcage into the floor. Pause before using the abdominals to draw the knees back to the starting position.

Technique tips

- Soften the ribcage as the knees lower.
- Roll the ribcage across the floor to draw the knees back.
- Range of movement is dependent on degree of control.

Tabletop exercises

True tabletop involves positioning the knees above the hips with spine in neutral. However, to ensure spinal safety at this stage, it is essential to use a modified version, known as 'imprinted' tabletop, where the knees remain over the chest and the lower back is in contact with the floor. This allows a safe margin of error so that participants will move into neutral rather than hyperextension if correct alignment cannot be maintained.

The following exercises are performed from the 'imprinted tabletop' position. Once stability has increased, they can all be progressed to a neutral tabletop position, but progress *must* be slow.

Moving into imprinted tabletop

- Recruit TrA and lift one foot off the floor, bringing knee up over chest.
- Allow the pelvis to tilt so the lower back makes contact with the floor.
- Lift the other knee up to join the first, maintaining back alignment.
- Draw knees together and ensure that the lower legs are parallel to the floor.

NB: To prevent hyperextension it may be necessary to use the hands to hold the first knee in position before lifting the second knee.

Figure 3.15 Toe touch

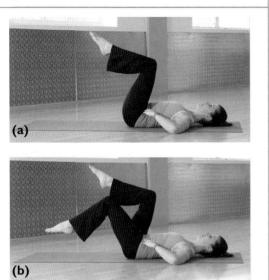

(a)

(b)

Technique tips

- Maintain 90° angle at the knee by keeping the lower leg lifted.
- Soften the ribcage as the leg lowers.
- Do not allow the pelvis to roll forwards as the leg lowers.
- Keep the upper body relaxed throughout.
- Avoid leaning on the elbows.
- Avoid gripping with the obliques.

NB: If discomfort is felt in the lower back, use your arms to hold the stationary knee towards your chest.

Progression

- When stability improves, this exercise should be performed from neutral, i.e. knees over hips, and neutral spinal maintained for the duration of the sequence.
- Perform with chest flye.

Toe touch

Preparation

In imprinted tabletop with elbows bent and fingertips resting on hip bones.

Action

Inhale to prepare and as you exhale recruit TrA and lower the right foot towards the floor, moving from the hip not the knee. Lower back should remain in contact with the floor. Return to the lifted position and repeat, using alternate legs. Begin with a small range of movement and increase it as stability improves.

Figure 3.16 Leg glide

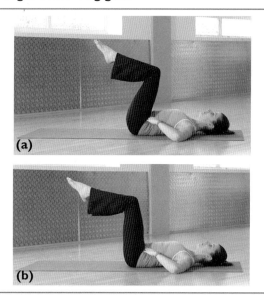

(a)

(b)

Leg glide

Preparation

In imprinted tabletop with elbows bent and fingertips resting on hip bones.

Action

Inhale to prepare and as you exhale recruit TrA and slowly glide your knees away from your chest, keeping the lower legs parallel to the floor and lower back on the floor. Pause very briefly, checking alignment, before returning to starting position. Begin with a small range of movement and increase it as stability improves. The further the legs are moved away from the chest, the more stability is required so begin with a small range of movement and increase it as stability improves. Increasing the range too soon will recruit the mobilising muscles.

Technique tips

- Soften the ribcage as the legs move away.
- Do not allow the pelvis to roll forwards with the legs.
- Keep the lower legs parallel to floor.
- Keep the upper body relaxed throughout.
- Avoid leaning on the elbows.
- Avoid gripping with the obliques.
- This exercise can also be performed with feet resting on a stability ball.

Progression

- When strength increases, this exercise can be performed from neutral. The movement should be very small, 3–6cm, with spinal alignment maintained.
- Perform with arm circle.

Caution: Stop immediately and review technique if discomfort is felt in the lower back.

Figure 3.17 Single leg stretch

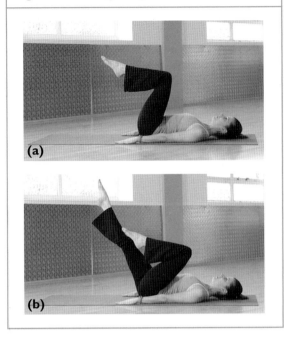

(a)

(b)

Technique tips

- Any outward movement of the leg challenges stability and should be adjusted as necessary.
- Soften the ribcage as the legs move away.
- Do not allow the pelvis to roll forwards with the leg.
- Avoid locking the knees.
- Keep the upper body relaxed throughout.
- Avoid leaning on the elbows.
- Avoid gripping with the obliques.

Caution: If discomfort is felt in the lower back, keep the top leg high and the bent knee in towards the chest. Taking the leg too low may cause the lower back to buckle away from the floor.

Adaptation

Keep one foot on the floor and perform in neutral alignment.

Single leg stretch

Preparation

In imprinted tabletop with elbows bent and fingertips resting on hip bones.

Action

Inhale to prepare and as you exhale recruit TrA and extend one leg towards the ceiling, drawing the other knee further into the chest. Continue with alternate legs, moving both simultaneously and keeping the lower back into the floor. Bending the top leg slightly will avoid pulling on the hamstrings. Once co-ordination and stability have been achieved, the top leg can be lowered a little way towards the floor (to approximately 60 degrees).

RECTUS ABDOMINIS

Why do you need to shorten RA?

The overstretched RA muscle must be shortened before strengthening can begin. If strengthening exercises commence before the muscles have realigned or before the re-education of TrA, doming will occur on engagement.

Which exercises will help to shorten RA?

- Posterior pelvic tilting in as many positions as possible, which will draw the two ends of the muscle closer together
- Working RA within its 'inner range', e.g. half roll back or curl-up with pelvic tilt

When can resisted RA work commence?

It is important to check the condition of RA to determine how far apart the two sides of the muscle are lying. This is done using the 'rec check'. Commencing resisted RA work with a wide separation will impair abdominal recovery (*see* page 52 for further discussion on resisted RA work). Results will depend on several factors: size of the baby, number of pregnancies, exercise history and the amount and type of exercise performed since delivery.

The 'rec check'

The following description is for self-testing of RA separation. Further guidelines follow for checking your client.

Preparation

Lie supine in neutral spinal alignment. Relax the abdomen and place two fingers of one hand immediately above the umbilicus, with the palm of the hand facing up towards sternum. Apply gentle pressure to the abdomen – long nails may be a hazard!

Action

Inhale to prepare and as you exhale recruit TrA and slowly raise head and shoulders off the floor, keeping gentle pressure on the abdomen with the fingertips. Hold, continuing to breathe, and register the sensation felt under the fingertips. Lower the head and shoulders with control, keeping the fingers in position.

Explanation

- As the head and shoulders lift, you should be able to feel two bands of recti muscle closing in around the fingers. They will feel like hard ridges on either side of the fingers, with the dip of the linea alba in the centre.
- If this cannot be felt, it may be necessary to curl up a little higher.
- If the gap between the two muscle bands appears to be wider than two fingers, repeat the test using three fingers.
- Repeat the test just below the umbilicus as the reading may be different.
- Check several times until you are sure of the result.

NB: Connective tissue between the two bands of recti muscle will still be stretched and weak so the fingers will sink deeply into the abdomen during this test.

Teaching the 'rec check'

When teaching this to a client, it is essential to explain clearly the purpose of the test and how the results will affect her recovery, as a hands-on experience like this may not be welcomed by some women.

It is helpful to explain the location of RA and the changes it has undergone during pregnancy. The explanation can be complemented by demonstrating with an *undone zip* (approximately 50cm long) showing the points of attachment of the muscle onto the pubis and sternum, and how the two sides stretch away from the midline as pregnancy increases. The zip can also be used to clarify how the shortening of these muscles encourages them back into correct alignment. This visual aid improves understanding of a rather complex concept. It is important that individuals understand exactly what they are feeling for, so that when the hard ridges of muscle butt against the side of the fingers they can distinguish between this and the soft, pliable centre. Re-testing at a later date is excellent confirmation of progress.

Some women may dislike pushing their fingers into their abdomen, particularly around the umbilicus, and may feel very sensitive about performing the test. Most women will want clarification of their findings, particularly those with minimal separation, as it will be more difficult to palpate. An instructor should always wait to be asked by the individual and avoid performing the check without gaining permission first. Perform the test by kneeling alongside the client, facing towards her to maintain eye contact throughout. In this position it is advisable for the instructor to have the soft pads of the fingertips facing towards the client's pubic bone.

How wide should the separation be?

By eight weeks in most cases it will have recovered to approximately two finger widths (2cm) apart at the umbilicus, and many women will find that recovery plateaus at this point (Coldron et al. 2007). If the gap is wider than this, the muscles can still recover, provided the correct exercises are performed. Even when fully recovered, the muscles will always lie slightly apart (approximately 1.5–2cm) but the difference will

Figure 3.18 a and b) Self-testing for RA separation, c and d) Instructor clarification

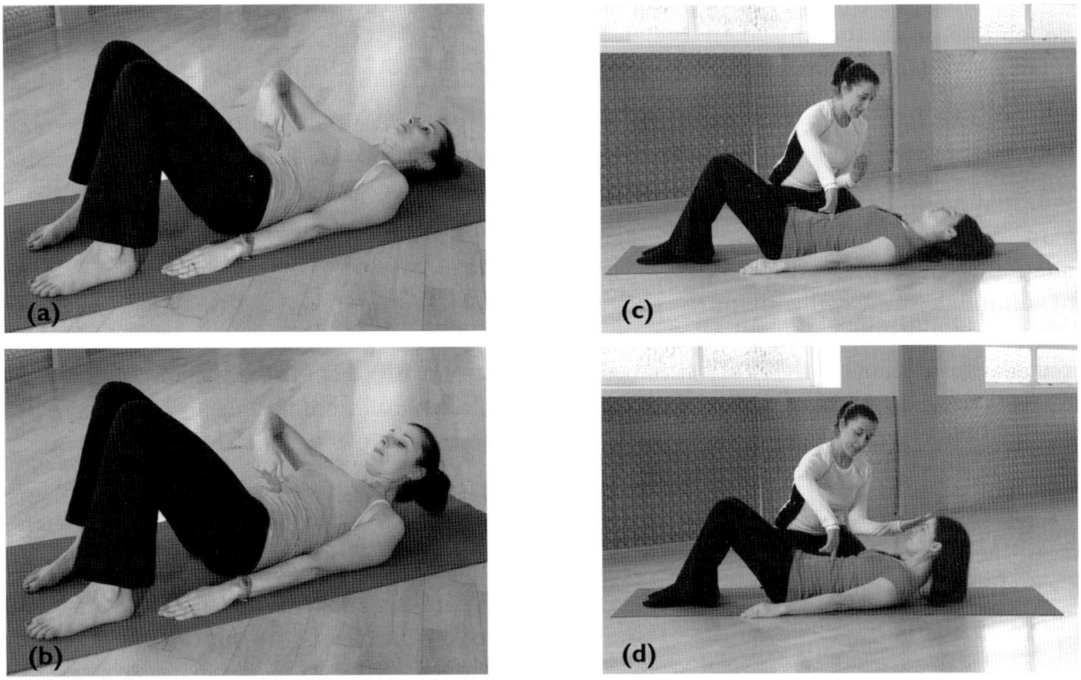

and shoulders. Keeping the buttocks lifted, hinge at the ribcage and lower slowly down to the floor, one vertebra at a time. Release and return to neutral spine. Encourage natural breathing throughout.

Technique tips

- Use the abdominals to create the movement.
- Try to separate each vertebra to make individual contact with the floor.
- Keep the weight on the upper part of the shoulder blades – do not lift onto the neck.
- Maintain alignment at the top of the move – keep the ribs down.
- Focus on the hinge of the ribcage at the beginning of the descent.
- Scoop in the abdominals to aid spinal flexion.
- Slow down through any tight areas to increase range of movement.
- Lengthen the tailbone away from the head as you lower.
- Draw shoulder blades down into the floor as you lower, to avoid hunching the upper body.

Caution: If gluteus maximus is weak, dominant hamstrings will grip to extend the hip and this may induce hamstring cramps.

Progressions of this exercise to challenge gluteus maximus are shown on page 118.

Kneeling pelvic tilt

Preparation

In four-point kneeling with spine in neutral alignment.

Action

Inhale to prepare and as you exhale recruit TrA and tilt the pelvis under, curling the tailbone to bring hips closer to ribs. Keep the elbows slightly bent to prevent them locking. Hold for a few seconds, continuing to breathe. Lower with control to the starting position, taking care not to let the back arch.

Technique tips

- Use RA to create the movement – avoid squeezing the buttocks.
- Focus on rib–hip connection.
- Lengthen tailbone away from head.
- Keep the shoulder blades sliding down.
- If you find this position uncomfortable due to tingling or numbness in the fingers, you could try resting your forearms on a chair.

Figure 3.21 Kneeling pelvic tilt

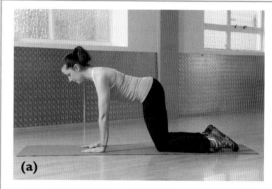
(a)

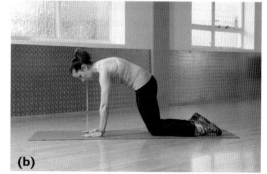
(b)

Figure 3.22 Kneeling pelvic tilt with head curl

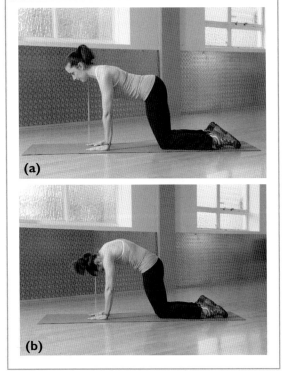

(a)

(b)

Figure 3.23 Seated pelvic tilt

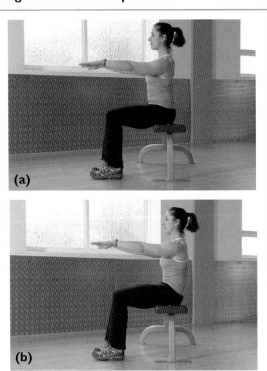

(a)

(b)

Kneeling pelvic tilt with head curl

In addition to shortening RA this is a great stretch for the spine.

As for kneeling pelvic tilt above, but taking the movement further by lifting and rounding the back towards the ceiling, drawing ribs closer to hips and curling the head under towards the pubic bone.

Seated pelvic tilt

Preparation

Seated on chair or floor in neutral alignment (*see* page 32), with hands holding lightly under thighs.

Action

Inhale to prepare and as you exhale recruit TrA and tilt the pelvis, scooping the abdominals and lifting the pubic bone up as you roll off your sit bones onto the upper part of the buttocks. Avoid using the arms for support. Pause, continuing to breathe. Return to upright seated position.

Figure 3.24 Head position when raising: a) correct, b) incorrect

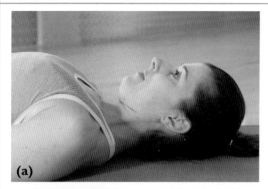

(a)

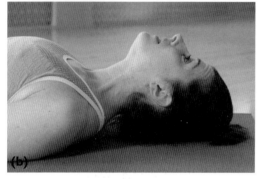

(b)

Technique tips

- Avoid leading with the shoulders.
- Use the abdominals to create the pelvic tilt.
- Think of lengthening while curling – avoid collapsing into the lower back.
- Focus on rib–hip connection.
- Create a C shape through the back (it may be necessary to squeeze the buttocks to achieve correct position).
- Release the shoulders and keep the head aligned.
- Return to upright seated position if the abdominals start to quiver.

Caution: If the abdomen begins to dome, return to the starting position and try again, ensuring TrA has been pre-engaged. If doming continues, reduce the range of movement. If discomfort is felt in the lower back, reduce the range of movement.

Progression

This can be developed into an inner range exercise – see below.

Inner range training for RA

Seated pelvic tilt

As above, but gradually increasing the length of hold to 30 seconds. Return to upright seated position if the abdominals start to quiver as this is an indication of overworking.

Progression

- Take away the hand support and extend your arms out in front at chest height. Range of movement may need to be reduced to maintain technique.
- Once this can be comfortably achieved increase the range of movement by curling back a little further.
- Hold in the rolled-back position and perform a few repetitions of the scissor arms exercise (*see* page 33).

Figure 3.25 Head and shoulder raise with pelvic tilt

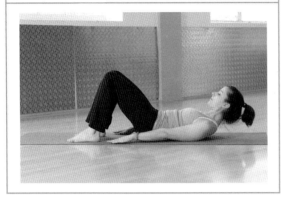

Head and shoulder raise with pelvic tilt

This exercise is the only resisted flexion exercise in the programme and has been included for RA shortening and inner range training only. Reasons for this are discussed later. Due to the technical difficulty of performing this exercise safely and effectively it is more suitable for 1–1 than group training. Head placement is another consideration.

Incorrect head position

Soreness and discomfort in the neck is frequently experienced with curl-ups and this can be attributed to weak neck flexors that have been compensated as a result of increased thoracic kyphosis. This is compounded by neck tension, experienced by many postnatal women, due to 24/7 baby care.

Overflexing the neck (chin tucked tightly into chest) or extending the neck (pushing the chin forwards) to try to assist the curling action creates further discomfort.

Correct head position

Keeping the head relaxed on the floor, lengthen through the back of the neck so that the chin draws down towards the chest but is not tucked tightly inwards. Slide the shoulders down your back, keeping the length through the back of the neck, as you curl the ribs towards the hips. An excellent aid is to hold the baby's squeaky toy under the chin without squeaking or dropping it; alternatively, placing the tongue on the roof of the mouth relieves stress to the neck flexors.

Preparation

Lie supine in neutral spinal alignment, with hands relaxed on the floor beside you. Lengthen the back of the head along the floor, drawing the head into correct alignment.

Action

Inhale to prepare and as you exhale recruit TrA, tilt the pelvis and curl your ribcage towards your hips, raising head and shoulders off the floor. Keep the head in line with the spine as you lift. Pause at the top then lower with control to neutral starting position.

Technique tips

- Think of creating the movement from the ribcage rather than the head and shoulders.
- Reach the arms towards the feet as you curl the spine.
- Keep the neck long and the shoulder blades down.
- Ensure that TrA is activated prior to lifting.
- Avoid gripping in the hips.
- Do not allow the back to overextend on release.
- Initially you may find it more comfortable to place a cushion underneath your head – move it away when you begin to feel stronger.

Caution: Curl up only to the point where the abdomen can be held in flat; if doming occurs the curl must be kept lower.

What's wrong with curl-ups?

While most women are desperate to start curl-ups as soon as possible, it should be explained they will not flatten the abdomen – and this is probably the reason they want to do them! Poor lumbopelvic stability results in increased IAP being exerted onto the abdominal and pelvic floor muscles during a curl-up, resulting in the abdomen being pushed out and/or the pelvic floor pushed down. O'Dwyer (2009) suggests that activities which increase the load on the PFM are completely inappropriate for women with dysfunctional PFM (*see* chapter 6 for further discussion).

What if lumbopelvic stability has been regained?

Once RA has shortened and regained strength in its inner range, strengthening exercises for RA and EO should be incorporated into functional movements that increase strength for activities of daily living (ADL). With the exception of getting out of bed, these muscles are not required for any other resisted supine activity so why train them in this position? Challenging the muscles in an upright position improves lumbopelvic stability, trains the whole body to

work as one integrated system and improves functional fitness.

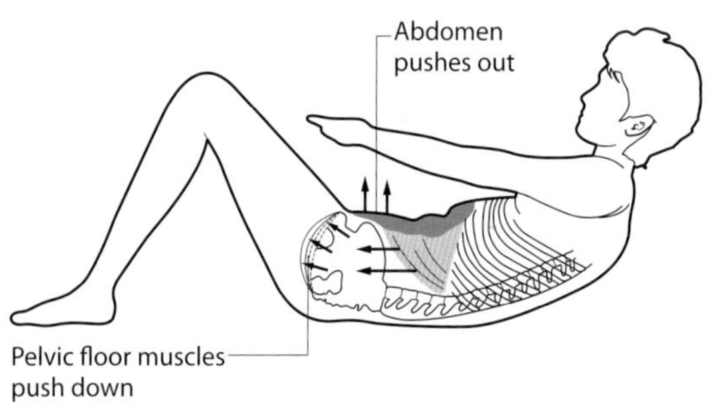

SUMMARY

- The rectus sheath is made from the aponeuroses of the three layers of abdominal muscle.
- The aponeuroses from each side join in the middle to form the linea alba.
- The abdominal aponeuroses are affected by relaxin, which allows the rectus abdominis to stretch and separate from the midline.
- Rectus abdominis may lengthen by approximately 20cm and the waistline may increase by approximately 50cm.
- The muscles begin to realign three to four days after delivery, but may take six weeks or longer to repair.
- Pelvic tilting and inner range training will assist RA shortening.
- TrA is a deep postural muscle and can only function at low intensities.
- Once fired up TrA should continue to work for the duration of that movement pattern.
- More difficulty recruiting TrA may be experienced after a caesarean delivery.
- Vigorous drawing in of the abdomen recruits other abdominal muscles.
- Constant reminders will encourage misrecruitment and should be avoided.
- Lumbopelvic stability should be regained with low-level exercises.
- High-intensity 'stability'-type exercises should be avoided until lumbopelvic support is established.
- Curl-ups are inappropriate for women with PFM dysfunction – 50 per cent of postnatal women!
- Challenging the abdominal muscles in functional positions is recommended.

Figure 3.26 Effects of curl-ups on poor lumbopelvic stability

Abdomen pushes out

Pelvic floor muscles push down

REFERENCES

Boissonnault, J.S. & Blaschak, M.J. 1988. Incidence of diastasis recti abdominis during the childbearing year. *Physical Therapy* 86: 1082–6

Boissonnault, J.S. & Kotarinos, R.K. In *Obstetics & Gynaecology Physical Therapy* Wilder, E. (ed.) (Oxford: Churchill Livingstone, 1988) 3: 63–82

Coldron Y., Stokes M.J., Newham, D.J. & Cook, K. 2007. Postpartum characteristics of rectus abdominis on ultrasound imaging. *Manual Therapy* 10: 1016

Commerford, M. 2008. The truth about transversus: Clinical application of the research. Lecture notes from presentation attended at University College London

Cresswell, A. 1993. Responses of intra-abdominal pressure and abdominal muscle activity during dynamic loading in man. *European Journal of Applied Physiology* 66: 315

Hodges, P.W. & Lee, L.J. 2009. Moving on from giving isolated core stability exercises. Seminar notes from presentation attended at University College London

Hodges, P.W. & Richardson, C.A. 1996. Inefficient muscular stabilization of the lumbar spine associated with low back pain: A motor control evaluation of transversus abdominis. *Spine* 21: 2640

Kendal, F.P., McCreary, E.K. & Provance, P.G. *Muscles: Testing and Function* 4th edn. (Philadelphia, USA: Williams & Watkins, 1993)

Lee, L.J. 2006. Is it possible to be too stable? *Orthopaedic Division Review* Nov/Dec

Lovering, R.M. & Anderson, L.D. 2007. Architecture and fiber type of the pyramidalis muscle. *Anatomical Science International* 83(4): 294–7

Morkved, S & Bo, K. 1996. The effect of post-natal exercises to strengthen the pelvic floor muscles. *Acta Obstetetricia et Gynaecologica Scandinavica* 75: 382–385

Myers, T. 1998. The abdominal balloon – Part 1: the dynamics of the abdomen (Body cubed series). *Massage Magazine* May/June

Norris, C.M. 2000. *Back Stability.* Leeds: Human Kinetics, 1

O'Dwyer, M. 2009. Hold it sister – The confident physio's guide to core and floor rehabilitation. Seminar notes from presentation attended at St Thomas' Hospital, London

Richardson, C.A. & Jull, G.A. 1995. Muscle control – pain control. What exercises would you prescribe? *Manual Therapy* 1: 2–10

Sapsford, R.R. 2008. Co-ordination of the abdominal and pelvic floor muscles. PhD Thesis, University of Queensland

Sapsford, R.R., Hodges, P.W., Richardson, C.A., Cooper, D.H., Markwell, S.J. & Jull, G.A. 2001. Co-activation of the abdominal and pelvic floor muscles during voluntary exercises. *Neurourology & Urodynamics* 20: 31–42

Sheppard, S., 1996. The role of transversus abdominis in postpartum correction of gross divarication recti. *Journal of Association of Chartered Physiotherapists in Women's Health* No. 79: 24–25

Stelzner, F., Beyenburg, S. & Hahn, N. 1993. Acquired disorders of peritoneal cavity muscles, abdominal wall denervation in pregnancy, denervation incontinence and continent and incontinent constipation. *Langenbecks Archiv fuer Chirugie* 378(1): 49–59

THE PELVIC FLOOR

4

THE STRUCTURE OF THE PELVIC FLOOR

The pelvic floor is a muscular platform at the base of the pelvis. Formed by a combination of muscles and fascia, it resembles an elastic sling at the pelvic outlet to support the pelvic and abdominal contents. Attached to the walls of the pelvis from the pubic bone at the front to the coccyx at the back, it consists of two halves joined in the middle to allow the urethra, vagina and anus to pass through. Superficial muscles form a figure eight around these openings. The pelvic floor comprises four layers:

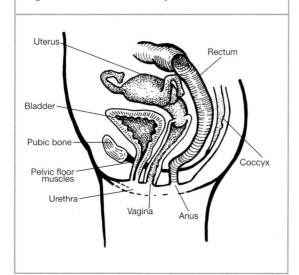

Figure 4.1 Side view of pelvic floor muscles

Uterus

Rectum

Bladder

Pubic bone

Coccyx

Pelvic floor muscles

Urethra

Vagina

Anus

1 The deepest is a layer of fascia located above the muscles themselves, which surrounds and suspends the organs and provides attachment for the pelvic floor muscles (PFM). This layer provides limited support and requires the assistance of the pelvic floor muscles when under pressure.

2 Levator ani is a group of muscles, forming the principal muscular layer, that inter-connect with the layers of fascia above and below. They form a muscular platform through which the urethra, vagina and anus pass. Levator ani assists with the sphincteric control of the bladder and bowel (Brook et al. 2008).

3 The perineal membrane is a dense triangular membrane situated towards the front of the pelvic floor. It connects the urethra and vagina to the walls of the pelvis. Made of fascia, it contracts reflexly to provide support when the levator ani muscles relax.

4 The superficial perineal muscles form the external genital muscles and are arranged in a figure eight around the openings – the anterior loop surrounds the urethra and vagina and the posterior loop surrounds the anus. These loops meet in the centre to form the perineum. Their function is mostly sexual as they offer minimal assistance to the continence mechanism.

Figure 4.2 Deep levator ani muscles

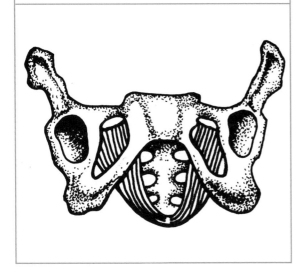

Figure 4.3 Superficial muscles of the pelvic floor

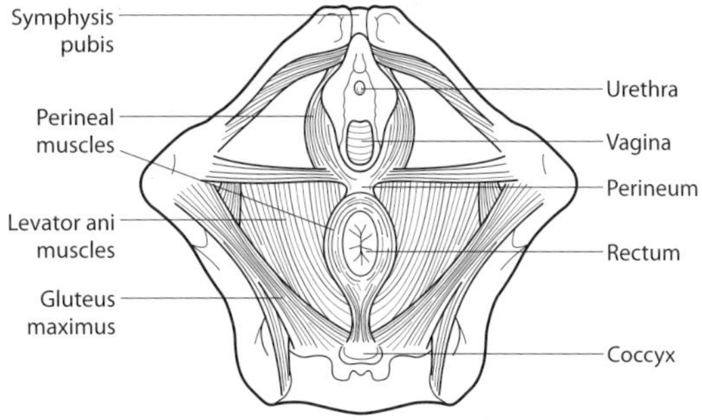

Symphysis pubis

Perineal muscles

Levator ani muscles

Gluteus maximus

Urethra

Vagina

Perineum

Rectum

Coccyx

FUNCTIONS OF THE PELVIC FLOOR

- Support the pelvic organs to prevent prolapse
- Promote urinary and faecal continence
- Stabilise the lumbar spine and pelvis
- Resist sudden rises in intra-abdominal pressure (IAP)
- Suppress sudden urge to void
- Inhibit bladder activity
- Help baby to turn during delivery
- Increase sexual satisfaction

Mechanics of continence

The bladder and PFM work together antagonistically: during voiding, the bladder, which is a muscular bag, contracts to expel its contents and the PFM relax; on completion of voiding, the PFM contract and the bladder relaxes to allow refilling. Continence is dependent on the amount of pressure exerted by the urethral sphincter to maintain closure and this must remain higher than the bladder pressure, both at rest and on physical exertion. The PFM contribute significantly to the continence mechanism, providing about one-third of urethral closing pressure (Rud et al. 1980)

Slow- and fast-twitch muscle fibres

Both slow- and fast-twitch fibres are found in levator ani (Jozwik & Jozwik 1998). Approximately 65 per cent of levator ani are slow-twitch (Gilpin et al. 1989) and thus perform a largely stabilising and supportive role. Engaged at lower levels they provide support for the organs, maintain the bladder neck at an optimum angle and inhibit unwanted bladder activity.

The fast-twitch fibres, accounting for approximately 35 per cent (Gilpin et al. 1989), are recruited during maximum activity to counteract rapid rises in IAP, e.g. due to a cough or sneeze, when they contract to lift the bladder neck higher into the abdominal cavity to prevent urine leakage.

As part of the inner unit of local stabilisers,

these muscles should automatically tense before movement of the arms or the trunk (Hodges et al. 2003).

CHANGES TO THE PELVIC FLOOR DURING PREGNANCY

Increased weight of the pregnant uterus, suspended by lax ligaments, exerts additional, progressive forces on the pelvic floor, which is already undergoing key changes as a result of increased relaxin production. The levator ani is encased between two layers of connective tissue, and its supportive role reduces as the muscles stretch beneath the heavy load; nerves activating these muscles may also be stretched. Tooz-Hobson et al. (2007) suggest that pregnancy itself increases the risk of stress incontinence, regardless of the type of delivery.

Collagen make-up determines the strength of connective tissue and this is genetic, so some women will be more at risk than others, i.e. a woman who experiences severe stretch marks, or is hypermobile, is more likely to have problems with her PFM. This is confirmed in a study by Eaves et al. (2006) who conclude that an intrinsic connective tissue abnormality is exacerbated, rather than caused, by pregnancy. It is not uncommon for women to suffer stress incontinence in late pregnancy because of these changes.

Effects of a vaginal delivery on the pelvic floor

A woman's first vaginal delivery causes muscle, fascial and nerve damage and it is likely that further damage will occur with future deliveries (Allen et al. 1990). During the second stage of labour all the layers of the pelvic floor must stretch to allow the baby to descend; quick progress down the birth canal or lack of elasticity

Figure 4.4 Levator ani muscles during delivery

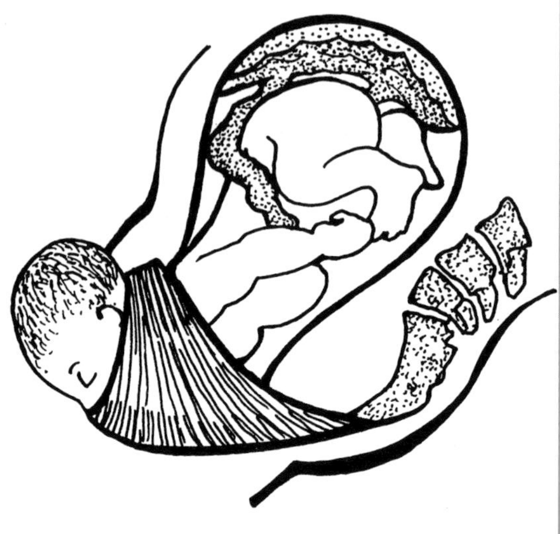

may cause a tear in one or more layers. Lien et al. (2005) suggest both the levator ani and urethral sphincter are stretched to the point of potential damage. The pudendal nerve, which activates the urethral sphincter, may also be overstretched.

Trauma to the perineum may occur through tearing or episiotomy. Pregnancy and childbirth are major contributory factors to PFM dysfunction (Freeman 2002). Following childbirth, a staggering 50 per cent of women have some degree of pelvic organ prolapse with symptoms of bladder and bowel dysfunction (Hagen et al. 2006).

Damage or weakness in one section of the inner unit will affect the action of the other components of the deep stabilising system, namely posture and respiration.

Figure 4.5 Effects of a vaginal delivery on the pelvic floor

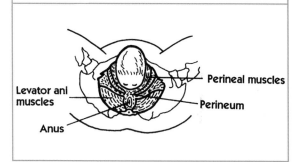

Levator ani muscles

Perineal muscles

Perineum

Anus

Episiotomy

An episiotomy is an incision in the perineum to enlarge the vaginal opening. No longer performed as a matter of routine, episiotomies are only usually required for assisted deliveries or to speed up delivery if baby is distressed.

Stitches

If the perineum has been cut in an episiotomy, or a tear continues to bleed, it will be repaired with stitches. Healing usually occurs within 10 days, but it may take up to six weeks for stitches to dissolve.

Caesarean delivery

Many women who deliver by caesarean section do not appreciate the need to continue PFM exercises postnatally. Although these muscles have not experienced the excessive stretching and trauma of a vaginal delivery, relaxin has still increased connective tissue elasticity and the muscles have supported the weight of the growing baby for nine months. A caesarean delivery following active labour may still incur levator ani damage. The case for pelvic floor exercises is strong, regardless of the delivery.

Stress incontinence

Stress incontinence is the involuntary loss of urine during physical exertion, e.g. coughing, sneezing, straining, lifting or jumping, and is not uncommon following childbirth. Like TrA, poor functioning of the PFM may be an issue of timing and therefore conscious activation, just prior to coughing or sneezing, will afford protection. Brooke et al. (2008) suggest this should become a lifelong habit.

Factors that may contribute to pelvic floor dysfunction

- Weaker collagen type.
- Overstretching of one or more of the muscle layers.
- Increased bladder neck mobility, which reduces the closing pressure exerted by the urethral sphincter.
- Overstretching of the pudendal nerve responsible for activating the PFM. Damage to this nerve will affect the ability of the muscles to contract. This is usually associated with a difficult labour, especially forceps delivery.
- Forceps delivery – a possible tenfold increase in PFM dysfunction (Kessel et al. 2001).
- Active second stage of labour longer than two hours.
- Lumbosacral and SIJ dysfunction (O'Sullivan et al. 2002).
- Baby weighing > 4kg.
- Race – Caucasian women may be more at risk than black women (Graham & Mallet 2001).
- Other reported risk factors include constipation, heavy lifting, inappropriate exercise, chronic cough, obesity, pelvic surgery, hormonal status and ageing (Brook et al. 2008).

Unfortunately many women believe it is a natural consequence of childbirth and often accept the condition. If exercises are not commenced or professional advice sought, the risk of short- and long-term problems increases. A regular programme of correctly performed PFM exercises may resolve this problem; if not, referral to a physiotherapist specialising in women's health may be necessary.

PELVIC FLOOR RECOVERY

The perineum may feel very sore and uncomfortable for many days after delivery, and it may be difficult to find a comfortable sitting position. Going to the toilet may be an uncomfortable and distressing experience so exercising that area may not be on the 'to do' list! Despite apprehensions, gentle exercise for the PFM promotes healing and aids recovery by increasing the flow of blood and nutrients for tissue repair and removing waste products. PFM exercises (PFME) will reduce the pain and discomfort experienced from a swollen and tender perineum, and assist the edges of a cut or tear to close together.

If the pudendal nerve has been overstretched during delivery, it will affect the messaging process from the brain to the PFM. Nerve stretch reduces muscle recruitment and recovery will be delayed until activation is possible. This may take approximately 6–8 weeks – longer in some cases, depending on the damage sustained. After this time, women may notice a sudden improvement in their condition, which may suggest to them that PFM strength has been gained and therefore a good reason to stop doing the exercises! However, this is only an indication that the muscles have been reactivated and it is important that a strength training programme commences from this point (*see* page 64).

Breastfeeding women may find it more difficult to strengthen the PFM in the first three months due to the suppression of oestrogen by the increased production of prolactin. Levator ani contains oestrogen receptors; low oestrogen levels associated with breastfeeding result in continued lack of muscular support.

When should pelvic floor exercises commence?

The body begins to repair itself immediately so to complement this, PFME should begin as soon as possible after baby is born – the sooner the better, ideally within 24 hours. Women who have never performed a PFME may experience difficulties recruiting stretched and weakened muscles and will need guidance and support to improve their confidence.

Effective teaching

Research by Bump et al. (1991) indicated that fewer than 50 per cent of women could perform a PFM contraction with just a verbal or written instruction. Given this, it is really important to spend time explaining the structure and position of the PFM before exercises are commenced; launching straight into it with no prior information will reduce effectiveness. While women will have been instructed to do these exercises after the birth, they may not be aware of their importance, particularly if everything seems to be working well with no leaks! A sore perineum may have discouraged commencement and the demands of a new baby take priority! Basic, user-friendly language, appropriate to the individual or group, is essential to focus attention on the position and functions of these muscles.

It may be helpful to use a model of a pelvis when explaining this, with both hands cupped underneath, to represent the muscles. Women must understand exactly what it is they are trying to do, particularly as there is no visible movement, and a clear explanation will help to build a better mental picture.

NB: Instructors *must* be able to contract their own PFM correctly before attempting to teach the procedure and should participate themselves while teaching it.

Two key factors – posture and breathing

As one of the muscles of the inner unit, co-ordination between the PFM and other three is vital to maintain lumbopelvic stability. A weakness in one causes adaptations to occur, with resulting inappropriate muscle substitution. Posture and breathing should be observed and corrected before attempting to locate and re-educate the PFM.

Posture

Adopting an upright posture in sitting and standing switches on the inner unit. Slumping or slouching shuts down TrA and the PFM and prevents the diaphragm from moving down during inhalation (O'Dwyer 2009). Encouraging good postural alignment at all times, not just while exercising, is the foundation of correct PFM (and TrA) recruitment.

Breathing

During inhalation the diaphragm moves down into the abdominal cavity; the PFM also move down but maintain support of the pelvic organs. During exhalation the PFM and diaphragm move up together (Myers 2000). Sapsford (2008) suggests PFM activity is greater during expiration than inspiration. This pattern *must* be established before PFME can be taught.

Poor breathing patterns restrict the movement of the diaphragm and this will affect PFM activation. Rib grippers demonstrate upper chest breathing that is noticeable in women with

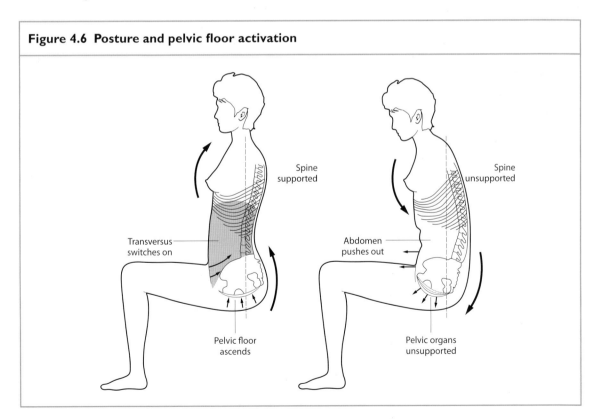

Figure 4.6 Posture and pelvic floor activation

Spine supported

Transversus switches on

Pelvic floor ascends

Spine unsupported

Abdomen pushes out

Pelvic organs unsupported

chronic chest disorders, such as asthma, or who are heavy smokers, as well as in women who constantly hold in their tummy using RA/EO. This mis-recruitment prevents the diaphragm from moving freely, as the ribs are 'fixed' and breathing becomes shallow, increasing tension in the neck and shoulders as the accessory breathing muscles overwork. O'Dwyer (2009) suggests this is also found in busy, high-achieving women who are always on the go, don't stop and relax and are unable to 'let go'. This could include a great deal of our clients – maybe ourselves too!

Many emotions are 'held' in the abdomen and pulling in the waist is part of the female psyche. If this 'holding' is done by RA/EO, the diaphragm, the PFM and TrA cannot function properly. Lee (2007(i)) confirms it is essential to teach correct diaphragmatic breathing to restore the function of the PFM. While this may seem a rather basic, time-consuming practice, it is an essential first stage of PFM retraining, which should not progress until women are competent.

Teaching correct breathing patterns

Wearing a tight bra or belt prevents the lower ribs from opening up during inhalation so it is important to feel comfortable.

- Position hands on lower ribcage, with fingers facing inwards.
- Inhale, taking the breath into the lower ribcage and abdomen, keeping RA/EO relaxed.
- Feel the ribs opening sideways and the abdomen swelling.
- As you exhale *relax* the ribcage and feel the diaphragm lifting up.

Relaxing the abdomen and letting it soften and swell may be very difficult for some women. After years of holding in, it may take time to feel comfortable with letting go. Encouragement,

empathy and praise are required. Practise in side/supine lying, seated and standing and keep checking for substitution.

If the PFM are working effectively, their recruitment should follow the diaphragm upwards on exhalation. If this does not occur automatically, these muscles need conscious activation. Always ensure that correct breathing is addressed before moving on to the recruitment stage.

Locating the right muscles

This is always a difficult one! With no visible movement and a very mild internal feeling, the biggest hurdle in PFM recruitment is locating the right bits! Stopping the flow of urine midstream is a technique frequently used to check the muscles are working effectively but this is an inappropriate way of testing muscle function and should never be practised (Walsh 2008). It confuses the bladder/PFM mechanism and increases the risk of urinary tract infections. More appropriate suggestions for correct recruitment include:

- Lying prone with one hand on the sacrococcygeal joint
- Leaning forwards in a seated position so the front of the PF is touching the chair
- Palpating on the bikini line
- Rising up onto, or scrunching the toes
- Inserting a finger into the vagina when showering
- Gripping partner's penis during intercourse (this method may be met with mixed reactions but is particularly helpful as feedback is available!)
- Sitting in front of a long mirror and observing if the waist inappropriately tightens

Some verbal cues are:
- Lift analogy – the PFM tighten as the lift doors close and draw up inside as the lift rises to the first floor
- Drawstring bag – imagine a string between pubic bone and tailbone, and between right and left sit bones, then lift up into the centre
- Lifting a tampon up inside
- Mini-tornado spiralling upwards
- Petals of a sunflower closing upwards

Approaches to teaching will vary and the selection of the most appropriate method will depend on the client/group, and the instructor's confidence and rapport with them. Confirmation of correct recruitment can only be made through a vaginal examination by a specially trained physiotherapist. Referral may be necessary for women who are experiencing problems.

Language

When teaching use clear, frank language, delivered with confidence. Avoiding essential terminology because of fear of embarrassment is unhelpful and will be counter-productive. Variations include:
- Stopping the flow of urine; passing water; having a pee/wee
- Stopping yourself passing/breaking wind
- Tightening/pulling up or in the vagina
- Gripping the penis/willy

RE-EDUCATING THE PELVIC FLOOR

Selecting an appropriate position in the early postnatal weeks is important for both comfort and achievement. Commence in side lying or supine positions as these reduce the load on the PFM – adopting neutral alignment if possible as this is more beneficial to recruitment (Sapsford et al. 2001).

Begin with the fast exercise (*see* page 62) as this is generally easier to do, particularly if there has been trauma to the area. Success with the fast exercise will increase confidence to try the slow one. Side lying may reveal a one-sided weakness, perhaps due to the lie or descent of the baby; however, exercising on both sides is recommended as there may be some crossover from the stronger side. Advise women not to leave it until the end of the day to do the exercise, as the muscles will be tired and substitution for muscles much more likely (*see* page 63).

The slow exercise should only be held for a few seconds initially, gradually increasing the length of hold. Attempting to hold for too long, too soon, results in the loss of activation and the unconscious 'fading' of the contraction. It is more effective to hold for a shorter period but still feel in control.

Once recruitment has been regained in an upright seated position, women should be encouraged to incorporate PFME into everyday activities, particularly when the muscles are loaded: sitting down, standing up, bending, lifting, carrying etc. In the learning stages, if women find PFME easier to do while standing they're probably doing them incorrectly and recruiting the assistance of RA/EO (O'Dwyer 2009). The presence of a horizontal crease in the abdomen and gripping under the ribs will confirm this – close observation is necessary.

NB: Practising PFME in the car at traffic lights is not such a great idea, as the seat of most cars encourages a slumped sitting position!

Training the PFM in functional positions is essential for improvement but the focus should be on achieving the best quality performance every time. Both slow and fast exercises should be performed in sets of low repetitions, frequently throughout the day. When coughing, sneezing or lifting, the PFM should always be consciously tightened to withstand the increased pressure. This counter-bracing action – known

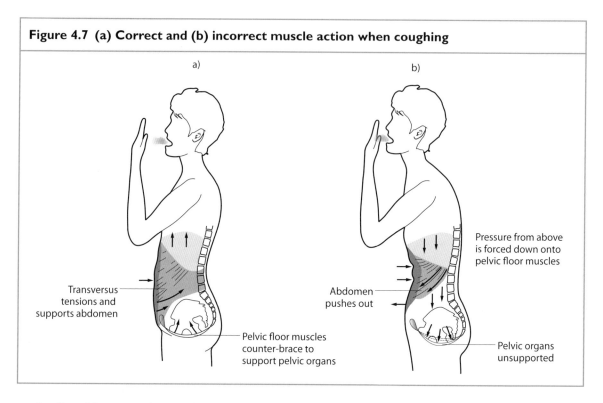

Figure 4.7 (a) Correct and (b) incorrect muscle action when coughing

a)

Transversus tensions and supports abdomen

Pelvic floor muscles counter-brace to support pelvic organs

b)

Pressure from above is forced down onto pelvic floor muscles

Abdomen pushes out

Pelvic organs unsupported

---

as the 'knack' – provides urethral support and may reduce leakage (Miller et al. 2001). Allowing the PF to be pushed down by the IAP increases the risk of prolapse. Strength training must not commence until the muscles can be correctly recruited, as this will just reinforce incorrect muscle recruitment and increase the pressure on the PFM.

Purpose of slow and fast exercises

Slow PFME will improve the resting tone of the muscle and this will maintain the bladder neck at its optimum angle. When IAP rises, the fast PFM contract to prevent urine loss. No matter how strong the reflex action is, if the bladder neck is not correctly aligned the fast-twitch PFM cannot prevent the loss of urine. The importance of working both types must be emphasised to provide optimum support.

There are variations of how these two exer-cises should be taught – the following are suggested.

Fast pelvic floor exercise

The fast exercise will help to strengthen the reflex action needed both to prevent the PF being pushed down when IAP rises and to close the bladder neck to prevent leakage.

Preparation

While this can be done in any position, it is advisable to start seated to check correct recruit-ment. Adopt neutral alignment.

Action

- Tighten and lift as high as possible in one quick contraction.
- Release immediately.
- Aim to repeat 8–10 times

NB: The aim of this exercise is to try to perform each contraction with the same speed and strength as the first. Keep repetitions low as fast-twitch fibres fatigue quickly.

Technique tips

- Exhale as you lift.
- Stay upright – do not bend at the waist.
- Avoid tightening the buttocks.
- Avoid pushing down on the release.

If difficulties are experienced, try placing hands firmly into the waist and cough slowly and strongly. Focus on the waistline pushing out to the side onto the hands.

Slow pelvic floor exercise

To retrain the stabilising function of the pelvic floor muscles the focus should be on obtaining a slow, gentle, submaximal contraction. Lee (2007(ii)) suggests concentrating on an activation that is more anterior (vaginal and urethral) than posterior (rectal).

Preparation

Assume any position – lying, kneeling, standing or sitting – in neutral alignment, with the feet slightly apart. On *every* occasion use the correct breathing pattern described previously.

Action

- Inhale as before.
- As you exhale draw the two sides of the PF in towards the centre.
- Wrap around the front as if you're stopping yourself having a wee.
- Lift up inside.
- Hold for a few seconds, continuing to breathe.
- Release and lower with control.
- Repeat 8–10 times.

NB: If the contraction fails after a few seconds and there is nothing left to release, the duration of hold should be shortened.

Technique tips

- Keep breathing throughout.
- Use a very slow, gentle drawing up action.
- See section below on muscle substitution for further comments.

Caution: Do not perform this exercise while passing urine.

> ### Important!
>
> During the fast or slow pelvic floor exercise, pushing down onto the PF instead of lifting is an inappropriate mis-recruitment that increases the risk of organ prolapse.

Substitution for weak stabilising muscles

Substitution occurs when the deep postural muscles fail to provide stability. The global muscles, RA/EO in particular, are then activated to help out and the body learns to cope this way every time support is needed. Continuing to use and tighten these muscles when the PF is weak or uncoordinated will force pressure downwards onto the PF and increase the risk of prolapse! (O'Dwyer 2009)

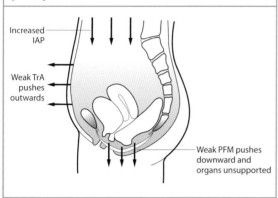

Figure 4.8 Pelvic floor depression and prolapse

Increased IAP

Weak TrA pushes outwards

Weak PFM pushes downward and organs unsupported

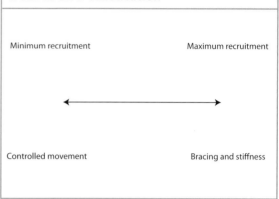

Figure 4.9 Increased pressure on the PFM from RA/EO substitution

Minimum recruitment   Maximum recruitment

Controlled movement   Bracing and stiffness

Failure of the stabilising muscles could be due to one or more factors:
- Incorrect timing (switching on too late)
- Lack of endurance
- Lack of strength

Unless the incorrect pattern of recruitment is stopped, the inner unit cannot resume control. The following coping strategies are frequently used and can be observed by an attentive instructor:
- Breath holding – EO are activated making it impossible to breathe.
- Narrowing or hollowing of the abdomen and a strong drawing down of the ribcage – involvement of RA and EO.
- Posterior pelvic tilt – RA and gluteus maximus activated (encouraging a slight medial rotation of the hip may reduce substitution).
- Squeezing inner thighs together – adductor activation (encouraging hip-width apart and no crossed leg sitting may reduce substitution).

Other considerations
- Poor posture is the No.1 cause of PF dysfunction (Sapsford et al. 2006). Correct standing and seated posture should be encouraged at all times but specifically reinforced while exercising the PFM.
- Allowing the abdomen to swell during recruitment suggests that the PF is being pushed downwards rather than lifted upwards.
- Lee (2008) suggests constipation may affect the ability of the PFM: if there are faeces in the rectum the PFM are required to generate more force.

EFFECTIVE TRAINING METHODS

It is vital that strength training for the PFM does not commence until they can be correctly recruited without substitution.

There are mixed opinions as to the most effective training methods but the general consensus seems to be that they should be realistic for the individual and performed regularly with thought and as much accuracy as possible. There is no limit to the number of repetitions to perform daily, provided the muscles do not fatigue. Morkved & Bo (1996) suggest an increase in strength can be achieved by performing three blocks of exercise daily which should aim to include 10 slow repetitions (progressing towards a 10-second hold) and 10 quick ones on each occasion.

As with any muscle training programme, overload is essential for muscle adaptation to occur. Use the 4 Rs to progress:

- **Rate:** Length of time held for / speed of contraction
- **Rest:** Length of time between repetitions
- **Repetitions:** Number of times performed
- **Resistance:** Side lying, bridge, supine, seated, standing, during squatting

Choose one method of progression at a time to promote success. Incorporate with ADL, particularly when lifting and carrying, and into an exercise programme.

How long should the exercises be continued?

Exercises for the PF should be continued for life! Unfortunately, it is around the three-month mark that many women stop doing PFME – if no problems have been experienced. They will have noticed an improvement (possibly nerve repair) and feel the muscles have recovered but strength has not been regained. Once learned, these exercises should be incorporated into their new lifestyle and continue as an essential daily undertaking.

Exercise and the pelvic floor

Activities that increase the load on the PFM are completely inappropriate for women with dysfunctional PFM (O'Dwyer 2009). These include high-impact work, curl-ups and lifting weights of any kind such as toddlers, buggies and car seats. To stabilise and support during higher loading, correct recruitment of the PFM is vital – without that, RA and EO will activate and increase the pressure on the PFM.

Once the PFM can be correctly recruited, and support regained, light weights can be used by women with previous experience; studio resistance classes should be avoided if inexperienced. The same principle applies to running: only those with previous experience and an appropriate low-level gait should resume, and even then it is not recommended before a minimum of 20 weeks post-birth. Further discussion on suitability can be found in chapters 9–11.

Abdominal exercises

If the PFM cannot be correctly recruited, the increased IAP created during abdominal work will be exerted downwards onto the vulnerable PFM, increasing the risk of prolapse. Vigorous resisted abdominal work should not be commenced until TrA and the PFM can be appropriately recruited and pelvic stability has been regained. Even then, its suitability is questionable!

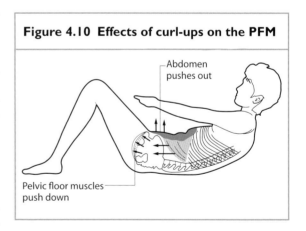

Figure 4.10 Effects of curl-ups on the PFM

Abdomen pushes out

Pelvic floor muscles push down

THE BREASTS

5

STRUCTURE

The breasts are modified glands that produce milk (Tortora & Grabowski 2003). They lie over pectoralis major and serratus anterior and are attached to them by a layer of deep fascia. They consist of glandular tissue and fat, embedded in a connective tissue framework known as suspensory ligaments, which run between the skin and deep fascia. The ligaments give support and shape to the breasts.

PREGNANCY CHANGES

With the rise in pregnancy hormones the breasts increase in size from as early as the first trimester. Increased levels of oestrogen allow fat to be deposited and, together with progesterone and relaxin, stimulate breast tissue growth. Relaxin also allows extensive branching and elongation of milk ducts and helps the nipples to enlarge (Bani 1997). Total breast weight may increase to approximately 800g. This large increase in size, together with the effects of relaxin on the supporting ligaments, leads to stretching of the breast tissue. Wearing a supportive bra during pregnancy will help to prevent excessive drooping, as will strengthening exercises for the pectoral muscles. In the third trimester a fourth hormone, prolactin, responsible for lactation, stimulates the production of colostrum, a yellowish fluid that may leak from the nipple and contains important nutrients for baby's first feeds.

POSTNATAL CHANGES

For the first few days following delivery the breasts continue to produce colostrum. It is low in fat but rich in proteins, carbohydrates and antibodies and easy for the baby to digest. Newborns' intestines are permeable and colostrum provides a barrier against foreign substances by sealing the lining. It is the fall in progesterone levels in the first 48 hours following delivery that triggers lactation.

Engorgement

When the milk comes in, on about day three or four after delivery, the breasts become engorged, i.e. hot, swollen and hard. This is due to an abundance of milk filling the ducts and an increased blood flow. Engorgement reduces as the baby begins to suck and this stimulates the continued production of prolactin. If breastfeeding is not commenced, prolactin levels return to normal within a few days and breast size slowly reduces. Engorgement can occur at any time during breastfeeding if supply exceeds demand for any length of time.

Hormonal changes related to breastfeeding

Oestrogen

As prolactin rises to support lactation, oestrogen levels are suppressed. Low oestrogen levels reduce the strength and support available from muscles and joint vulnerability continues.

Low oestrogen levels suppress ovarian function, which will reduce the likelihood of the menstrual cycle returning – although it does not give complete protection against further pregnancies! Suppressed ovarian function incurs several physiological changes similar to those of the menopause (Cunningham et al. 1997). These include hot flushes, night sweats, reduced vaginal secretions and reduced emotional stability. The most dramatic side effect is the quick and significant loss of bone mineral content: the loss averages about 5 per cent during the first three months (Little et al. 1993). This is because oestrogen is the essential element needed for maintaining bone density. It works in three key ways:

- Maintains the correct balance of bone formation and resorption
- Helps the body absorb calcium from the intestines
- Reduces calcium loss through the kidneys

The absence of oestrogen has a much greater effect on bone mass than do exercise and calcium intake: if the last two help maintain bone density by a factor of two, then oestrogen helps by a factor of 10 (Otis and Goldingay 2000). Breastfeeding women need around 1000mg of calcium per day and this should be available in a balanced diet. Women who are averse to dairy products, or do not eat a balanced diet, should refer to their healthcare provider for advice on supplementation. An adequate level of Vitamin D is also essential to facilitate calcium transfer from the intestines to the bloodstream and also to reabsorb calcium from the kidneys, preventing its loss in the urine. Outdoor walking should be encouraged, as sunlight provides a natural source of vitamin D.

Breastfeeding and bone mineral loss

Despite the rapid loss of bone mineral content in the first three months of breastfeeding, studies by Sran (2006) indicate that bone density is usually recovered within six months of finishing breastfeeding. The study also suggests that there is no additional loss if breastfeeding continues longer than six months, and that there is no difference between women after four+ pregnancies and those after two or fewer pregnancies.

Prolactin

Prolactin levels vary during the first three months after delivery and are determined by the frequency of suckling:

- During the first week there is a slight increase with suckling.
- Between two and twelve weeks, levels increase 2–3 times and regular suckling incurs a further 10- to 20-fold increase.
- After three months, baseline prolactin levels are similar to those of non-lactating women and do not rise significantly with suckling (Blackburn 2003). Reduction of prolactin levels allows oestrogen to rise and the consequential return of the menstrual cycle.

Dopamine

Dopamine, a neurotransmitter, is responsible for the flow of information across the brain and is associated with memory, attention span, processing and mood. Prolactin suppresses dopamine production and this may explain the postnatal 'baby brain' that many women can relate to. Loss of concentration and forgetfulness can also be attributed to the constant multitasking required of a new mum.

Empathy and consideration are important when training this client group as they will need clear explanations, technique reminders and lots of positive encouragement. Cardiovascular exercise increases dopamine release.

POSTURAL CHANGES

The increased size and weight of the breasts may pull the spine forwards; this, together with poor positions often adopted for feeding, may cause stress and discomfort to the cervical and thoracic spine. Correct posture should be adopted at all times, with particular emphasis on an extended, upright spine with shoulders relaxed (*see* chapter 1). Women who were previously quite small-chested may feel self-conscious about their new development but should be encouraged to keep the chest lifted to maintain correct postural alignment. Although information is given to new mothers regarding positions for feeding, they are not always practical to adopt, especially if baby is particularly fractious or having problems latching on to the breast. Poor feeding positions will increase the stress to the spine and create tension and aching in the neck and shoulders, which, if such positions are repeatedly adopted, may cause a great deal of discomfort. The correct posture for feeding is discussed in the Appendix.

EXERCISE AND BREASTFEEDING

Exercise and bone mineral loss

Regular weight-bearing activities and resistance training are strongly recommended to increase muscle mass and to support weakened structures. Recent studies by Lovelady et al. (2009) suggest that resistance and aerobic exercise may slow down bone loss during lactation!

Bone loading

Bone loading activities are essential but these must be over and above the regular level of activity undertaken to produce change. The key mechanical stresses on a bone are those that result from the pull of the skeletal muscles and the pull of gravity. The amount of force the body exerts on the ground is equal and opposite to the reaction force of the ground. The greater the force into the ground, the greater the effect on bone loading. It does not mean that postnatal women need to do high-impact work to recover bone density, as this is inappropriate for a multitude of reasons previously discussed, but careful selection of activities that increase the load to the bone without compromising other structures is recommended.

Use of variable directions is an important aspect of bone loading but as forward moving creatures we perform limited movements in a sideways, backward or diagonal direction. As bone density changes are specific to the site of strain, repetitive movements that are forwards travelling will load the bone in the same way. Multi-directional activities incorporating unfamiliar patterns of weight distribution are far more beneficial and appropriate to postnatal women and this should be considered when designing a postnatal programme.

Exercise and milk production

Studies by Carey & Quinn (2001) suggest that changes in lactate levels of breast milk only occur following maximal intensity exercise and this may affect infant acceptance of post-exercise breast milk. However, the authors agree there are flaws in this research and infant refusal of post-exercise breast milk may have been linked to other factors. In the absence of specific evidence it would seem that moderate-intensity exercise with good hydration will not affect the quality and quantity of breast milk. It is unlikely postnatal women would feel comfortable pushing themselves any harder.

Advice varies on the amount of fluid a breastfeeding woman should be drinking, apart from 'drink to thirst'. A common recommendation is to drink a glass of water with meals and whenever she breastfeeds (Montgomery 2002). There are no published guidelines on fluid intake during exercise, although Clapp (2002) suggests low fluid intake is directly associated with poor performance in both exercise and breastfeeding. Dewey et al. (1994) suggests that women who exercise and breastfeed frequently do not increase fluid intake sufficiently. The best way of monitoring this is for women to check the colour of their urine – the clearer it is, the better hydrated they are.

Breastfeeding and weight loss

Breastfeeding uses an average of 500 calories per day and appetite generally increases in response to this. Fat utilisation increases and this will assist weight loss, particularly if combined with moderate exercise and sensible eating. Drastic dieting or repeated sessions of very intense exercise may significantly reduce milk quality and quantity, or its production may cease completely.

EXERCISE CONSIDERATIONS

Feed before exercising

It is essential to feed or express milk before exercising to decrease the load and reduce leakage. Large, full breasts will feel uncomfortable if squeezed or bumped and vigorous, large-range arm movements may promote milk flow. A small amount of leakage may still occur during exercise even if a feed isn't imminent – mums are advised to wear breast pads.

What type of bra should be worn?

The breasts need stabilisation and support during exercise so a good bra is essential to prevent overstretching of the breast tissue. While a nursing bra is very convenient for feeding, it does not provide sufficient support for large moving breasts. A sports bra is recommended as it is designed to absorb shock and reduce the bounce of the breasts during physical activity (this could be worn over the top of a nursing bra if necessary). Wide shoulder straps help to distribute the weight across the shoulders more evenly and this will help prevent neck, shoulder and upper back pain. A deep band underneath the cups will provide good support – underwired bras should be avoided. Tight-fitting elasticated sports tops, which compress the breasts into the chest wall, may constrict the milk ducts and lead to mastitis.

Range of movement

To maintain comfort, a reduced range of movement may be necessary for some arm exercises. Elbow alignment may be difficult to maintain and consideration should be given to the fact that breast tissue also extends into the armpit. With the continued effects of reduced joint stability associated with breastfeeding, modifications are essential – body positioning and joint alignment should not be compromised in the desire to achieve results. Movements should continue within the regular range until breastfeeding ceases.

Body positioning

The breasts may feel extremely uncomfortable for most women when exercising in a prone position. For others, this position may be tolerated for short periods, provided feeding is not imminent. Rolled up towels placed above and below the breasts may reduce some of the pressure but this should be monitored as it may hyperextend the spine. Alternative positions or equipment should be used where possible, or commencement postponed until the prone position is comfortable. A forwards leaning position or four-point kneeling may cause additional drag and discomfort to heavy breasts. Stretches for the pectoral muscles should be performed with the abdominals pre-activated and the ribcage drawn down to prevent hyperextension.

SUMMARY

- Prolactin rises to support lactation, causing oestrogen to fall.
- Reduced oestrogen causes significant bone mineral loss.
- Calcium intake should be around 1000mg per day.
- Prolactin suppresses dopamine, which is a neurotransmitter.
- Total breast weight may increase up to approximately 800g during pregnancy.
- Large breasts will affect posture and may stress the spine.
- Poor posture and feeding positions may cause tension in the neck, shoulders and upper back.
- Feed before exercising to reduce the weight of the breasts.
- A good supporting bra is essential.
- Vigorous arm movements may cause the breasts to leak.
- Range of movement in the upper body may need to be reduced.
- Alternative positions may be necessary for breast comfort.
- Regular weight-bearing exercise is essential to increase muscle mass and support weakening bones.
- Ground reaction force is an essential factor in bone loading.

- Multi-directional activities are most appropriate.
- Moderate-intensity exercise and good hydration will not affect the quality and quantity of breast milk.
- Regular and plentiful intake of fluids is essential to avoid dehydration.
- Approximately 500 additional calories per day are required to maintain an adequate supply of milk.
- Breastfeeding increases fat utilisation, which may assist weight loss.

REFERENCES

Bani, D. 1997. Relaxin: A pleiotropic hormone. *General Pharmacology* 28(1): 13–22

Blackburn, S. 2003. *Maternal, fetal and neonatal physiology*. Oxford: Saunders

Carey, G.B. & Quinn, T.J. 2001. Exercise and lactation: Are they compatible? *Canadian Journal of Applied Physiology* 26(1): 55–74

Clapp, J.F. 2002. *Exercising through your pregnancy*. Nebraska, USA: Addicus Books Inc., 76

Cunningham, F.G., Macdonald, P.B., Gant, N., Gilstrap, L.C., Hankins, G.D.V. & Clark, S.I. (eds.) 1997. *Williams Obstetrics* 20th edn. Connecticut, USA: Appleton & Lange, 533–46

Little, K.D., Clapp, J.F. & Gott, P.D. 1993. Bone density changes during pregnancy and lactation in exercising women. *Medicine and Science in Sports and Exercise* 25(suppl. 1): 154

Lovelady, C.A., Bopp, M.J., Colleran, H.L., Mackie, H.K. & Wideman, L. 2009. Effect of exercise training on loss of bone mineral density during lactation. *Medicine and Science in Sports and Exercise* 41: 1831–1977

Montgomery, K.S. 2002. An update on water needs during pregnancy and beyond. *The Journal of Perinatal Education* 11(3): 40–2

Otis, C. & Goldingay, R. 2000. *The Athletic Woman's Survival Guide.* Leeds: Human Kinetics

Sran, M. 2006. Pregnancy and lactation associated osteoporosis. Lecture notes from presentation for The Guild of Pregnancy & Postnatal Exercise Instructors, London

Tortora, G.J. & Grabowski, S.R. 2003. *Principles of Anatomy and Physiology.* New Jersey, USA: John Wiley & Sons Inc.

- Keep the car seat close to you when lifting and carrying.
- Take particular care with domestic chores such as unloading the dishwasher/washing machine.
- Pace activity levels by incorporating short breaks into the day to avoid overdoing it.

See Useful Contacts for websites of PGP support groups offering further advice.

During pregnancy, women may have been advised to avoid opening the legs excessively and take care when getting in/out of car/bed. Continuing to over-protect the pelvis in this way may prolong tension in the adductors (Stuge 2009): postnatal women should be encouraged to move as 'normally' as comfort allows.

Exercise advice

The following should be considered:
- Exercising the adductor muscles – these muscles are likely to be very tight, so gentle stretching is more appropriate.
- Exercises for the abductor muscles – non-weight-bearing exercises are more suitable.
- Cross-trainers and steppers involve the repeated shift of body weight from one foot to the other – alternative equipment is recommended.
- Faster walking pace may bring on discomfort.
- Sidestepping action should not be taken too wide – even then it may be uncomfortable.
- Movements performed on one leg require close observation to ensure that weight is lifted out of the supporting hip – alternatives may be necessary.
- Rocking the hips excessively from side to side should be avoided.
- Breaststroke leg action during swimming may be uncomfortable.
- Seated stretch for the gluteals is particularly suitable as it also lengthens the adductors – if performed correctly it also puts the pelvis into good alignment.
- Avoid overdoing it – consider FITT.

Coccygeal pain

The coccyx articulates with the sacrum at the sacrococcygeal joint, where a small amount of movement occurs. As the baby travels down the birth canal, pressure is exerted on the coccyx, which may be pushed backwards causing bruising and inflammation. Women who have had a previous injury to their coccyx, from falling or slipping, are more at risk during a vaginal delivery. The resulting pain can be severe and incapacitating, and will make sitting extremely difficult. Straining on the toilet may also be very uncomfortable.

What can be done to help?

Sitting, particularly on hard surfaces, will be impossible and alternative positions, such as side lying, may need to be found for feeding. To reduce the pressure on the coccyx in a seated position, relief may be gained from sitting on a 'valley' cushion or inflatable head support often used as a travel pillow (*see* Useful Contacts for details of valley cushion suppliers). A swimming ring may be useful to sit on in the bath but is not recommended for long periods of sitting. Reducing the pressure on the coccyx enables good postural alignment to be maintained and reduces the tendency to want to lean forwards. Leaning back will cause pain! Drinking plenty of fluids to maintain hydration and regular walking may help to prevent constipation.

Exercise and a damaged coccyx

Floorwork will pose the greatest difficulties. It may be extremely uncomfortable, or even impossible, to lie supine in neutral alignment, and it may be necessary to tilt the pelvis posteriorly to lift the coccyx and reduce pressure on the area. Seated floor positions, such as hamstring and adductor stretches, may need alternatives, and any seated exercise that involves rolling off the sit bones, e.g. seated pelvic tilt, should be eliminated from the programme until the condition improves. The recumbent bike may also be inappropriate.

Knee pain

Softening of the articular cartilage of the patella may occur during pregnancy as a result of connective tissue changes. Reduced ligamentous support of the pelvic joints may alter the Q angle of the femur at the knee; this will affect the function of the quadriceps group and may create an imbalance in the lateral and medial thigh. Weight gain and altered posture will also increase the stress to the knee joint. Pain or aching will be felt in the front of the knee when it is flexed (such as when sitting, squatting or standing up) and is accentuated when walking downstairs. The increased need to bend, squat or kneel down while caring for baby may exacerbate this condition.

Exercise and knee pain

Most activities involve knee flexion at some stage, and it would be impossible to eliminate the action completely. However, activities involving repetitive knee flexion, e.g. step training or cycling, should be substituted by a more comfortable activity. Alternatives may need to be found if kneeling positions are uncomfortable, although this is less common. Increasing the strength of the quadriceps, particularly vastus medialis, will help to provide support around the knee joint and rebalance muscular strength in the quadriceps group (*see* 'Seated leg extension', page 117).

Backache

This is a very common postnatal complaint which may, to varying degrees, affect up to 50 per cent of postnatal women, many of whom were not affected during pregnancy. The lingering effects of relaxin on spinal stability continue into the postnatal period, and the increased size of the breasts and poor feeding positions place further stresses on the thoracic and cervical areas. Tight back extensors, weak gluteals and increased thoracic stiffness from pregnancy posture will contribute greatly to this. Weak, stretched abdominal muscles may be unable to maintain the correct tilt, and the constant bending and lifting, necessary for everyday baby care, will challenge reduced lumbopelvic stability. Discomfort may be experienced in all areas of the spine although the lumbar region tends to suffer most. Tiredness and fatigue associated with a new baby should also be considered as a contributory factor to the general aches and pains frequently experienced.

What can be done to help?

Postural correction plays an essential role in postnatal back care. Body positions should be carefully revised for correct standing and sitting, particularly during feeding, and good techniques adopted for lifting and carrying baby (*see* chapter 1 and Appendix). Exercises to increase lumbopelvic stability are vital (*see* chapter 2). Daily mobilising activities for the thoracic and lumbar spine, e.g. trunk rotations, hip circles and knee lifts, will help reduce stiffness together with stretches for the trapezius, latissimus dorsi, gluteals, hamstrings, hip flexors and piriformis (*see* chapter 8). Women should be encouraged to rest whenever possible, preferably not in a seated position, as this increases spinal pressure. Adopting positions in which the spine is supported, e.g. lying supine on a firm surface with legs bent up and resting on a chair or sofa, will enable the tight back muscles to relax.

Forearm, wrist and hand pain

Problems with the forearm, wrist and hand are not uncommon for postnatal women and tend to occur around six months after birth. This could be attributed to a combination of factors: connective tissue changes in the absence of relaxin, i.e. increased joint stiffness as a result of reduced joint laxity, and inflammation of the joints as a result of overuse with 24/7 baby care. In both conditions described below, sufferers may have difficulty caring for their baby.

Carpal tunnel syndrome

Carpal tunnel syndrome is caused by the compression of the median nerve as it passes through the narrow tunnel of bones in the wrist. During pregnancy it is related to increased levels of oestrogen, causing water retention; postnatally it may be an overuse condition causing inflammatory responses. Studies by Snell et al. (1980) suggest the condition seems to be related to breastfeeding hormonal changes, in that symptoms resolve within a few weeks of stopping breastfeeding. Tingling and numbness is experienced in the thumb, index and middle fingers.

Tendonitis

Inflammation of the tendons of the wrist flexors and extensors may occur as a result of overuse from repetitive movements. Manifesting in the thumb, wrist or elbow, pain is associated with grasping, twisting and holding actions – all required for babycare. Sudden intense pain, aggravated by repeated gripping, particularly in the thumbs, may be experienced. Anecdotally, this condition also seems to be related to breastfeeding hormonal changes although no evidence is currently available to support these claims.

What can be done to help?

With both conditions the alignment and position of the wrist is an important factor. Excessive and repetitive wrist flexion should be avoided wherever possible, and the adoption of a different hand position to support baby, particularly during feeding, may be helpful. Hooking the thumbs under baby's armpits when lifting will increase the strain on this joint. Finger and wrist mobility exercises, with the hands in an elevated position, may help reduce joint stiffness, as will stretching the muscles in question.

When walking with the buggy, negotiate bends with a wide sweep to prevent excessive rotation of the wrist/forearm and avoid over-gripping the buggy handle. Pushing the buggy with one hand, for example while talking on the phone or holding a toddler's hand, should be avoided wherever possible. Referral to a physiotherapist specialising in women's health may be necessary.

Exercise and wrist/forearm problems

Weight-bearing positions that require flexion of the wrist, e.g. four-point kneeling, may be extremely uncomfortable or in some cases impossible. Placing a rolled up towel under the heel of the hand may reduce discomfort if wrist flexion is a problem. Correct joint alignment is essential when using resistance equipment; lifts that require the arms to be in a downward position may be painful and induce loss of sensation in the fingers. Particular care should be taken when using resistance bands, as wrist/forearm alignment is easily compromised. Wrapping the bands around the hand is also inappropriate. Grip strength may be affected, particularly if the thumbs are sore – care and attention should be given to the use of all resistance equipment.

PELVIC FLOOR PROBLEMS

The PF is composed of muscles, nerves and connective tissue; damage to any of these structures has implications for its function.

Factors which may contribute to PFM dysfunction

- Weaker collagen type.
- Overstretching of one or more of the muscle layers.
- Increased bladder neck mobility, which reduces the closing pressure exerted by the urethral sphincter.
- Overstretching of the pudendal nerve responsible for activating the PFM. Damage to the pudendal nerve will affect the ability of the muscles to contract. Associated with difficult labour, especially forceps delivery.
- Forceps deliveries – a possible tenfold increase in PFM dysfunction (Kessel et al. 2001).
- Active second stage of labour longer than two hours.
- Lumbosacral and SIJ dysfunction (O'Sullivan et al. 2002).
- Baby weighing > 4kg.
- Race – Caucasian women may be more at risk than black women (Graham & Mallet 2001).
- Other reported risk factors include constipation, heavy lifting, inappropriate exercise, chronic cough, obesity, pelvic surgery, hormonal status and ageing (Brook et al. 2008).

Some problems may be resolved with correct and regular performance of PFME; others will need referral to a physiotherapist specialising in women's health or referral to a GP for medical intervention. For this reason only basic guidelines are given here.

Stress incontinence

This is the most common type of incontinence and the only one discussed in this book. Stress incontinence in postnatal women is the consequence of overstretched muscles and/or nerves within the PF musculature, which cannot activate or provide sufficient support when IAP rises. The PFM provide about one third of urethral closing pressure and a reduction in this support, together with increased mobility in the bladder neck, may result in a small leak of urine on exertion, e.g. coughing, sneezing, laughing, lifting, jumping or running.

What can be done to help?

Working 1–1 with a client provides an excellent opportunity to discuss these, very personal, issues. While this information may not be disclosed in the initial screening process, open discussion with women should be encouraged to establish if additional help is required. Very often women will assume it is a natural consequence of childbirth and may accept the situation; frequently they are too embarrassed to ask for help. This is confirmed in a study by Mason et al. (2001) who found that women with stress incontinence were reluctant to seek help, even though they were often inconvenienced and troubled by the condition.

It must never be assumed that women know how to activate their PFM correctly. Research by Bump et al. (1991) indicated that fewer than 50 per cent of women could perform a PFM contraction with just a verbal or written instruction. With this evidence in mind it is really important to start with the basics of posture and breathing as these are the two key factors involved in correct PFM recruitment, and these points may never have been addressed before (*see* page 59). Once posture and breathing has been established, a clear explanation of location and function should be given, using language appropriate to the client. Taking the time to do this, perhaps at the expense of other components of the workout, will greatly benefit the majority of women.

Teaching women to counter-brace the PFM just prior to a cough or sneeze – a manoeuvre known as the 'knack' – may reduce stress incontinence and retrain the fast-twitch fibres to work in an anticipatory role. A study by Miller et al. (2001) confirms that a PFM contraction in preparation for, and through, a cough can provide urethral support during stress.

It is important to note that the maintenance of good hydration levels is vital during exercise. Sufferers may deliberately avoid fluids prior to and during exercise for fear of an accident but dehydration increases the concentration of urine and further irritates the bladder. Regular sips of water should be encouraged.

Exercise and stress incontinence

Activities that increase the load on the PFM are completely inappropriate for women with dysfunctional PFM (O'Dwyer 2009). This includes high-impact work, curl-ups and lifting weights of any kind, such as toddlers, buggies and car seats.

SOFT-TISSUE AND OTHER PHYSIOLOGICAL PROBLEMS

Diastasis recti

During pregnancy the abdominal muscles undergo a tremendous amount of stretching, facilitated by increased connective tissue elasticity. The two bands of recti muscles, which previously lay parallel, stretch away from the midline to allow space for the growing uterus. A study by Boissonnault & Blaschak (1988) reported separation occurring in 27 per cent of women in the second trimester and 66 per cent of women in the third trimester. The umbilicus appears to be the weakest point, with a higher percentage of separation occurring here than above or below (Gilleard & Brown 1996). It is thought that the structure of the abdominal aponeuroses below the umbilicus provides additional reinforcement, as all layers of the aponeuroses pass over the top of RA at this level. The

size of the separation can vary from a small gap, measuring 2–3cm wide and 2–5cm long, to a larger gap of 12–20cm wide and possibly extending almost the length of the linea alba (Polden & Mantle 1990).

What are the risk factors for diastasis recti?

Lo et al. (1999) suggest these factors:
- Multiparity (having had more than one child)
- Maternal age > 34 years
- Larger babies
- Greater weight gain
- Caesarean section
- Multiple gestation

Other studies have found that women providing childcare are also at risk: increased strain on the weakened abdominal wall and use of the Valsalva manoeuvre when lifting may contribute to widening of the separation (Barton 2004). Candido et al. (2005) suggest there may be a reduced risk of diastasis recti in women living in extended family settings, which may protect them from strenuous work and childcare during pregnancy. Lack of regular exercise during pregnancy has also been identified as a risk factor.

How long does recovery take?

By eight weeks most women will have recovered to approximately 20mm (two finger widths) apart at the umbilicus and for many women recovery will plateau at this point (Coldron et al. 2007). By the time women are ready to return to exercise following their postnatal check-up, separation will probably have reduced. However, this should not be assumed and testing for abdominal separation is essential (see page 44). Separation of more than two fingers at this time does not necessarily indicate a permanent problem, provided the correct exercises are given (see below).

What advice should be given for continuing separation of less than two finger widths?

Exercises to increase lumbopelvic stability (*see* chapter 3) are vital and should not be missed out because the client (or instructor) finds them boring or considers them a waste of time! These exercises involve gentle TrA recruitment in association with low-level limb movement to encourage the stabilising muscles of the inner unit to work together as one. If taught correctly they will help to increase the tone of the linea alba and improvements can be palpated with regular rec checks – the fingers will not sink as far as before and a degree of resistance will be provided by the linea alba. Improvement may be slow but perseverance from both parties will pay off! Pelvic tilting exercises, in as many positions as possible, are also important to shorten the lengthened RA.

NB: High-intensity isolated 'abdominal hollowing' exercises are inappropriate as they will recruit EO, which pull on the weakened linea alba and exacerbate the problem.

Important!

In cases where the abdomen remains distended and pendulous, it is essential that the woman is referred to a physiotherapist specialising in women's health or advised to visit their GP for medical attention.

Lifestyle advice

Correct upright posture should be encouraged during everyday activities, as this will assist recruitment of the deep stabilising muscles. Guidelines should be given for care of the abdominals when getting up from a lying position: roll onto one side before sitting up, and reverse the process when lying down. Gentle recruitment of TrA prior to bending will ensure activation of the stabilising muscles to provide support. Lifting toddlers and heavy shopping, moving furniture, pushing a heavy trolley etc. should all be avoided wherever possible. If these cannot be prevented, recruitment of TrA and PFM prior to the movement will provide stability to the linea alba as the global stabilisers (RA/EO) activate to assist with higher level loading.

Exercise and diastasis recti

The following should be avoided:
- Resisted flexion – curl-ups!
- Specific exercises for the oblique muscles due to their insertion into the aponeurosis.
- High-intensity, so-called 'stability' exercises, often performed on uneven surfaces such as a ball. The 'plank' exercise also falls into this category.
- Over-enthusiastic tightening and gripping of the abdomen in the mistaken belief that isolated TrA exercises will flatten the tummy!
- Any exercise or activity that involves strong rotation or side flexion.
- Movements that stretch the abdominals.
- Exercises in the four-point kneeling position may be unsuitable due to increased load on the weakened structure.
- Any exercise that causes doming.

Perineal trauma

It has been suggested that as many as 85 per cent of women suffer some form of perineal trauma following a vaginal birth, with 60–70 per cent requiring stitches (Kettle 2006). Short-term complications include pain, infection and haemorrhage; long-term effects include incontinence of urine, faeces or wind, prolapse and painful intercourse. Presentation of any of the above long-term effects need referral to a specialist physiotherapist in women's health.

The perineum may be sore for some days or

even weeks following delivery, and many women have difficulty finding a comfortable sitting position – making feeding more difficult. Discomfort may be experienced from bruising, episiotomy or a tear that has not repaired well, either due to poor stitching leading to lumpy scar tissue, or because of infection.

What can be done to help?

PFME are invaluable in assisting the healing process, although many women may be apprehensive about doing these if they are feeling uncomfortable. Pain may be more severe with the first contraction but should decrease with repetition as the swelling is reduced. Increased blood flow to the damaged tissue speeds up the healing process, removing waste products from the area and helping the edges of a cut or tear to close together. The use of ice packs on the perineum may help to reduce swelling and supporting the area during a bowel movement is recommended. It is vital that the PF is contracted prior to coughing, sneezing or lifting to counter-brace the rise in IAP.

Prolapse

A prolapse is the bulging of the bladder or rectum through the wall of the vagina, or the descent of the uterus into the vagina. These pelvic organs are held in position by ligaments and the PFM are sandwiched between layers of connective tissue, all of which are affected by changes in collagen structure during pregnancy. Further weakening or damage may occur during labour and/or delivery. Bulging of the bladder against the front wall of the vagina is the most common postnatal prolapse condition, although a prolapse of the rectum may sometimes occur. Uterine prolapse is more often associated with the menopause, when low levels of oestrogen decrease the elasticity of the vaginal walls. Other causes of a prolapse may be contin-

uous heavy lifting (as in strength training), incorrect performance of PFME (i.e. bearing down rather than contracting and lifting up), chronic constipation or a chronic cough. Some degree of prolapse is seen in 50 per cent of women who have given birth (Hagen et al. 2006).

What are the symptoms of a prolapse?

A dragging sensation, or a feeling of something 'coming down' in the vagina, low backache and heaviness. This feeling is experienced when standing and becomes progressively more uncomfortable through the day. It appears to go away when lying down.

What can be done to help?

PFME may delay or even prevent the need for surgery to repair a prolapse, as correctly activated strong PFM will help to support the pelvic organs. It is important to maintain good hydration levels and avoid caffeine, which may irritate the bladder. As with stress incontinence, activities that increase the load on the PFM are completely inappropriate, so lifting or pushing a resistance should be avoided. Professional advice should be sought at the earliest opportunity.

Haemorrhoids

Haemorrhoids are varicose veins in the anal passage. Relaxation of the smooth muscle tissue of the intestines during pregnancy results in increased fluid absorption and the slowing down of the passage of waste material through the gut. This often leads to constipation, and the consequent straining to move the bowels causes ballooning of the veins in and around the anus. Haemorrhoids may appear for the first time after delivery as a result of pushing in the second stage of labour and may cause extreme discomfort, e.g. itching around the anus and pain/bleeding when passing motions. Constipation will compound this problem.

What can be done to help?

The use of ice packs may ease the pain and reduce the swelling, and frequent pelvic floor exercises will also be beneficial. The advice for constipation given in the next section can also be helpful here.

Constipation

Constipation is extremely common during the early postnatal weeks, probably due to:
- Fear of pain or tearing in the pelvic floor during bowel movements.
- Dehydration caused by loss of fluids in breast milk or a reduction in fluid intake due to fear of leakage.
- Weak abdominals reducing IAP.
- Inactivity – regular exercise aids digestive system function.
- Insufficient fruit and fibre because of concerns over the effects on breast milk.
- Never finding a quiet moment to go to the toilet – sometimes baby has to come too!

What can be done to help?

Gentle cardiovascular exercise such as walking is highly recommended as it increases the heart rate and promotes circulation. Women should be advised to drink plenty of water and increase their intake of fibre. Toilet habits are also important: squatting puts the bowel in the right position to empty but sitting on a toilet reduces the mechanical advantage of this position. Slumping in the lower back will close the anal sphincter and this needs to be relaxed and open for efficient emptying. Raising the feet onto a small stool and leaning forwards onto the knees may be helpful. Straining and breath holding will increase the pressure on the PFM. Supporting the perineum with a pad of toilet paper may be helpful during bowel movements to prevent the perineum bulging.

Varicose veins

Varicose veins may occur during pregnancy, normally in the legs. They are caused by the relaxing effects of progesterone on the walls of the veins and the resulting inefficiency of the vein valves in closing and securing a one-way flow of blood back to the heart. This causes the veins to swell and the legs to feel tired and heavy. After delivery there is often an improvement in the severity of this condition, although appropriate leg care should still be continued.

What can be done to help?

Avoid sitting with crossed legs or kneeling back on the heels as this will compress the veins and further reduce blood flow. Sitting with legs supported in a raised position whenever possible may reduce discomfort.

Exercise and varicose veins

Exercises that increase the blood flow through the calves are recommended, as the pumping action of the muscles will assist blood flow back to the heart. Walking is the ideal activity for its additional benefits, but standing calf raises and seated ankle circles with legs raised are equally helpful. Motionless standing should be avoided.

Mastitis

Mastitis is an inflammation of the breast tissue that arises when milk is not emptied from the breast as quickly as it is produced. There are several possible causes of this:
- Blocked duct
- Incorrect positioning of the baby
- Pressure from the hands holding the breast to feed
- Tight seat belt
- Wearing a tight bra

Cracked nipples can also lead to infection.

> ## Important!
>
> Mastitis causes the breasts to become red and lumpy and extremely painful. In this case the woman may feel feverish and quite ill, and is advised to visit her GP immediately to seek medical attention. Unless the problem is treated quickly, a breast may become infected and develop an abscess, which may require surgical intervention.

Exercise following mastitis

Prone positions are inappropriate due to the pressure on the breasts. An adapted front lying position, with elbows supporting the upper body to keep the breasts off the floor, is also unsuitable as it may hyperextend the spine. Since the breast tissue extends into the armpit, many arm movements may cause discomfort. A good supportive bra is essential but it should not be so tight that it constricts the breasts excessively.

EMOTIONAL PROBLEMS

Women may experience a variety of emotions following birth and some are a normal part of early motherhood whilst others are more serious.

- **Baby blues** is a mild, transitory condition experienced in varying degrees by 70–80 per cent of women (ACOG 2009). It generally commences a few days after delivery and lasts only a few days. Women feel emotional and upset, crying for seemingly trivial reasons, and may find it impossible to cheer up.
- **Postnatal depression** is a mild, moderate or severe condition that can affect up to 10% of new mothers (ACOG 2009). It can occur at any time within the first year but seems to be most common when the baby is between four and six months old. It may come on gradually over a period of time or start suddenly. Postnatal depression has many symptoms, often beginning in a similar way to baby blues but developing to more severe feelings of anxiety and stress. Some women suffer panic attacks and feel restless and irritable; they may become very anxious about their own and their baby's health, while others may show very little interest in the baby. Some women feel guilty that they are not coping as well as they think they should.
- **Puerperal psychosis** is a much more serious condition that requires immediate psychiatric intervention and hospitalisation. This condition requires specialist treatment and is beyond the realms of this book.

Postnatal depression

What are the causes?

The birth of a baby is a deeply emotional time, bringing intense feelings of joy as well as overwhelming anxiety. The causes of postnatal depression can be numerous and complex and may include physical, emotional and lifestyle issues. Gjerdingen & Dwenda (2003) suggest that women with a history of previous postnatal depression have a 50–60 per cent risk of a subsequent episode. Physical factors relate to the dramatic change in the level of hormones after delivery together with the demands of round-the-clock baby care and diminishing energy levels. Other factors may relate to a major role change: loss of independence, freedom and income accompanied by a feeling of isolation and lack of adult conversation. Concerns relating to the health of the baby, breastfeeding, change in body shape etc. will all contribute to emotional change at a time when a woman is already feeling exhausted and vulnerable.

Exercise and postnatal depression

The case for the use of exercise in reducing the symptoms of postnatal depression is strong! Several studies suggest that exercise is as effective as psychotherapy and antidepressant therapy in treating mild to moderate depression (Manber et al. 2002). Sampselle et al. (1999) suggest that exercise positively influences mood in new mothers. A study on the effectiveness of a pram walking exercise programme in reducing depressive symptoms in postnatal women (Armstrong & Edwards 2004) suggests that it is not just improvements in fitness that have an impact on depression. Exercise can serve as a distraction, or time out from daily hassles and stressful situations, and improve self-esteem with the acquisition of a new skill. It has many positive effects but the difficulties lie in actually getting these women to participate!

The added advantage of a specific postnatal exercise session is that it provides an opportunity to meet other new mums, share experiences and concerns and find that much needed empathy and support from others. Easy to follow, safe and effective exercise designed specifically to meet their postnatal needs will improve physical fitness and may reduce feelings of fatigue and help rebuild self-confidence.

Cardiovascular exercise is particularly beneficial as it promotes production of endorphins, the body's natural opiates, which together with other hormones are believed to improve mood. Increased blood flow occurring with CV exercise also helps to disperse adrenalin, which builds up when the body is stressed Encouragement and praise from the instructor is essential as well as increased sensitivity when correcting poor performance. A period of structured relaxation is suggested although, if anxiety levels are high, individuals may find it almost impossible to relax. In such cases it is useful to provide opportunities to rest without a specific relaxation section – i.e. movements and/or positions that help to ease tension and promote calm. Relaxation techniques are discussed in chapter 13.

It is important to remember that postnatal depression is an illness and women will need support from appropriate professionals. Help and support is available and referral back to their GP for advice may be necessary (*see* Appendix for details).

SUMMARY

- PGP occurs in one in five pregnant women.
- Increased levels of relaxin are not generally the cause of PGP.
- There is no apparent relationship between pain and increased range of movement in the pelvic joints.
- PGP may be associated with inappropriate muscle recruitment patterns.
- A damaged or bruised coccyx may prevent some floor positions being adopted.
- Changes in the Q angle of the knee and repetitive bending may induce knee problems.
- Correct posture can reduce backache.
- Exercises to improve lumbopelvic stability may reduce back pain.
- Forearm, wrist and hand pain is associated with excessive repetitive movements.
- Tingling and numbness in the fingers may limit the amount of weight-bearing exercises that can be performed. Grip strength may also be affected.
- Wide separation of RA may continue for some time into the postnatal period. Resisted abdominal work should be avoided and appropriate instructions for exercise transitions given.
- Damage to muscles, nerves and connective tissue of the pelvic floor has implications for its function.

- Counter-bracing the PFM on exertion may protect against stress incontinence.
- Seated positions may be uncomfortable for a sore perineum.
- High-impact exercise, curl-ups and lifting weights of any kind is inappropriate for dysfunctional PFM.
- Gentle CV exercise and increased fluid intake will help improve constipation and haemorrhoids.
- Painful breasts following mastitis may reduce the range of movement in the upper body and prevent some positions being adopted.
- Exercise is beneficial for reducing symptoms of postnatal depression.

REFERENCES

ACOG (American College of Obstetricians and Gynaecologists) 2009. Postpartum depression. Patient education leaflet

ACPWH (Association of Chartered Physiotherapists in Women's Health) 2007. Pregnancy-related pelvic girdle pain. Guidance booklet for health professionals

Armstrong, K. & Edwards, H. 2004. The effectiveness of a pram walking exercise programme in reducing depressive symptomatology for postnatal women. *International Journal of Nursing Practice* 10: 177–94

Barton, S. 2004. The postnatal period. In: Mantle, J., Haslam, J. & Barton, S. (eds.) *Physiotherapy in Obstetrics and Gynaecology* 2nd edn. Oxford, Butterworth Heinemann

Boissonnault, J. & Blaschak, M.J. 1988. Incidence of diastasis recti abdominis during the childbearing year. *Physical Therapy* 86: 1082–6

Brook, G., Coldron, Y., Evans, G., Gulliford, G.J., Hawkes, R., et al., 2008. Chapter 5: Physiotherapy in women's health. In: Porter S. (ed.) *Tidy's physiotherapy* 14th edn. Oxford, Churchill Livingstone

Bump, R.C., Hurt, G.W., Fantl, J.A. & Wyman, J.F. 1991. Assessment of kegal pelvic muscle exercise performance after brief verbal instruction. *American Journal of Obstetrics and Gynaecology* 165: 322

Candido, G., Lo, T. & Janssen, P.A. 2005. Risk factors for diastasis of the recti abdominis. *Journal of the Association of Chartered Physiotherapists in Women's Health* 97: 49–54

Coldron, Y., Stokes, M.J., Newham, D.J. & Cook, K. 2007. Postpartum characteristics of rectus abdominis on ultrasound imaging. *Manual Therapy* 10: 1016

Elden, H., Hagberg H., Olsen, M.F., Ladfors, L. & Ostgaard, H.C. 2008. Regression of pelvic girdle pain after delivery: Follow-up of a randomized single blind controlled trial with different treatment modalities. *Acta Obstetricia et Gynecologica Scandinavica* 87(2): 201–8

Gilleard, W.L. & Brown, J.M.J. 1996. Structure and function of the abdominal muscles in primigravid subjects during pregnancy and the immediate postbirth period. *Physical Therapy* 76(7): 750–62

Gjerdingen, D. 2003. The Effectiveness of Various Postpartum Depression Treatments and the Impact of Antidepressant Drugs on Nursing Infants. *Journal of the American Board of Family Practitioners* 16: 372–82

Graham, C.A. & Mallet, V.T. 2001. Race as a predictor of urinary incontinence and pelvic organ prolapse. *American Journal of Obstetrics and Gynaecology* 185(1): 116–20

Gutke, A., Ostgaard, H.C. & Oberg, B. 2006. Pelvic girdle pain and lumbar pain in pregnancy: A cohort study of the consequences in terms of health and functioning. *Spine* 31: 149–55

Hagen, S., Stark, D., Maher, C. & Adams, E. 2006. Conservative management of pelvic organ prolapse in women. *Cochrane Database of Systematic Reviews* 18(4) CD003882

Hansen, A., Jensen, D.V., Larsen, E.C., Wilken-Jensen, C., Kaae, B.E., Frolich, S., et al. 2005. Postpartum pelvic pain – the 'pelvic joint syndrome': A follow-up study with special reference to diagnostic methods. *Acta Obstetricia et Gynecologica Scandinavica* 84: 170–6

Kessel, K.V., Reed, S., Newton, K., Meier, A. & Lenz, G. 2001. The second stage of labour and stress urinary incontinence. *American Journal of Obstetrics and Gynaecology* 105: 1300–7

Lee, L.J. 2009. Can you be too stable? Notes from presentation attended at City University, London

Lo, T., Candido, G. & Janssen, P. 1999. Diastasis of the recti abdominis in pregnancy: Risk factors and treatment. *Physiotherapy Canada* 44: 32–7

Manber, R., Allen, J.B. & Morris, M.M. 2002. Alternative treatments for depression: Empirical support and relevance to women. *The Journal of Clinical Psychiatry* 63(7): 628–40

Marnach, M., Ramin, K., Ramsey, P., et al. 2003. Characterization of the relationship between joint laxity and maternal hormones in pregnancy. *Obstetrics and Gynecology* 101(2): 331–5

Miller, J.M., Perruchini, D., Carchidi, L.T., Delancey, J.O.L. & Ashton-Miller, J. 2001. Pelvic floor muscle contraction during a cough and decreased vesical neck mobility. *Obstetrics and Gynecology* 97(2): 255–60

NICE Guidelines 2006: CG37 Postnatal care of women and their babies, National Institute for Health and Clinical Excellence, www.guidance.nice.org.uk, 100

O'Dwyer, M. 2009. *Hold it sister – The confident girl's guide to a leak-free life.* Queensland, Australia: Redsok

O'Sullivan, P.B., Beales D., Beetham, J.A. et al., 2002. Altered motor control strategies in subjects with sacroiliac joint pain during the active straight leg raise test. *Spine* 27(1): E1

Polden, M. & Mantle, J. 1990. *Physiotherapy in Obstetrics and Gynaecology.* Oxford, Butterworth-Heinemann

Sampselle, C.M., Seng, J. & Yeo, S.A. 1999. Physical activity and postpartum well-being. *Journal of Obstetric and Gynaecological Neonatal Nursing* 28(1): 41–9

Snell, N.J.C., Coysh, H.L. & Snell, B.J. 1980. Carpal tunnel syndrome presenting in the puerperium. *Practitioner* 224: 191–3

Stuge, B. 2009. Stabilising exercises – how and for whom? Seminar notes from presentation attended at the Conference of the International Organisation of Physical Therapists in Women's Health, Lisbon

Vleeming, A., Albert, H.B., Ostgaard, H.C., Sturesson, B. & Stuge, B. 2008. European guidelines for the diagnosis and treatment of pelvic girdle pain. *European Spine Journal* 17(6): 794–819

REFERENCES

National Institute for Health and Clinical Excellence (NICE) 2006. CG37 Routine post-natal care of women and their babies. http://guidance.nice.org.uk

SELECTED POSTNATAL EXERCISES

On the days immediately following birth the introductory exercises for learning to recruit the deep stabilising muscles correctly can be commenced, e.g. adopting correct spinal alignment, breathing techniques and locating TrA and the PFM (*see* chapters 2, 3 and 4). Spending time on these exercises in the early days is time very well spent!

The mobilising exercise at the beginning of this chapter can also be included and will help to loosen the body and reduce stiffness. From about day eight, depending on how the woman is feeling, some of the Level 1 lumbopelvic stability exercises can be introduced. Even at this very basic stage, correct technique is paramount, but without the guidance of an instructor good performance may be difficult.

When women have been given the go-ahead to exercise following a satisfactory postnatal check-up, instructors should always go back to the basic exercises described above – regardless of the type of exercises these women have been doing. Always check with them first as it is possible some women will have been recommended to do curl-ups! The race to flatten the tummy will increase their focus on this area but they should be reminded that correct performance of any exercise will enhance this!

Good posture and alignment should be adopted at all times.

STANDING POSTURE

- Stand, with the feet hip-width apart (underneath ASIS).
- Spread weight equally between both feet.
- Distribute weight evenly between big toe, little toe and heel.
- Soften the knees and align them over the ankles.
- Find your neutral pelvis (*see* page 8).
- Slide your shoulders down and relax your elbows.
- Lengthen your tailbone towards the floor, keeping your buttocks relaxed.
- Extend your spine upwards.

Figure 8.1 Correct posture

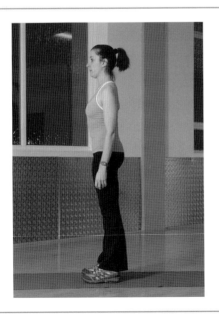

- Lengthen the neck, keeping the chin parallel to the floor.
- Look straight ahead.

NB: Postnatal women will often adopt a wider stance as they feel their hips have widened during pregnancy. This should be corrected if the correct stance is still comfortable.

Important!

Gently drawing in the abdomen to recruit TrA should be cued at the beginning of each exercise and normal breathing encouraged throughout. It is not necessary to give constant reminders to activate TrA – once they have been recruited they should continue to work for the duration of the exercise.

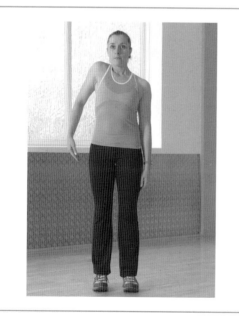

Figure 8.2 Shoulder circle

EXERCISES FOR MOBILITY

Shoulder circle

Purpose: to mobilise the shoulder joint.

Preparation

Stand in correct upright posture, arms relaxed by sides.

Action

Gently draw in the abdomen and slowly circle the shoulders forwards, upwards, backwards and downwards in a large exaggerated way, maintaining spinal alignment. Repeat slowly several times.

Technique tips

- Emphasise the backward and downward movements.
- Keep both hips facing forwards.
- Maintain upright stance.
- Keep the knees soft.
- Keep the movement slow and controlled.

Figure 8.3 Side bend

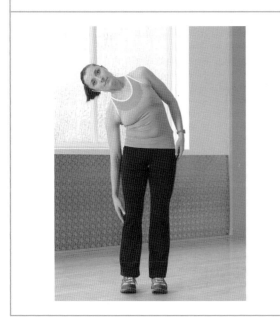

Action

Gently draw in the abdomen and bend slowly sideways from the waist, reaching down towards the floor. Return to the lifted position and stand tall. Repeat on alternate sides.

Technique tips

- Bend directly to the side – do not lean forwards or backwards.
- Keep the weight central throughout – avoid pushing the hips out to the side.
- Bend as far as is comfortable.
- Lift up on the underneath side – avoid collapsing.
- Lengthen the spine in the upright phase.
- Keep the movement slow and controlled.

Side bend

Purpose: to mobilise the spine.

Preparation

Stand in correct upright posture, with arms relaxed by sides. Standing with feet too wide will encourage hip sway to the opposite side and reduce the degree of lateral spinal flexion.

Figure 8.4 Trunk rotation

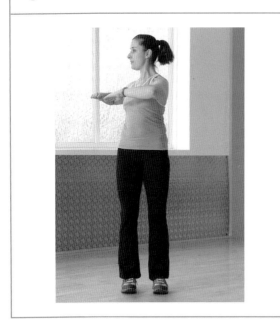

Action

Gently draw in the abdomen and, keeping the knees and hips facing forwards, slowly rotate the upper body around to one side. Return to the central position before rotating to the other side. Repeat as required.

Technique tips

- Knees and hips should remain square to the front.
- Draw the shoulder blades down.
- Lengthen the spine as the upper body rotates.
- Pause to check upright standing posture before each rotation.
- Keep the movement slow and controlled.

Caution: Allowing the knees and hips to rotate may be damaging to the knees and lower back. It also defeats the purpose of the exercise!

Trunk rotation

Purpose: to mobilise the thoracic spine, which becomes very stiff during pregnancy.

Preparation

Stand in correct upright posture. Bend the elbows and lift the arms to chest height.

Figure 8.5 Hip rotation

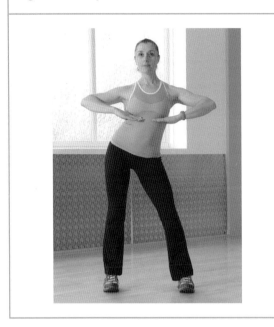

Action

Gently draw in the abdomen and, keeping the knees soft and spine long, slowly move the hips around in an exaggerated circle. Repeat as required before changing direction.

Technique tips

- Movement should occur below the hands – avoid moving the upper body.
- Keep the chest lifted and spine long.
- Weight should remain centred between the feet throughout.
- Keep the movement controlled and continuous.
- Encourage full and free range of movement.

Hip rotation

Purpose: to loosen the lower back.

Preparation

Stand in correct upright posture, with feet wider than hips and hands on the lower ribcage.

Figure 8.6 Heel toe

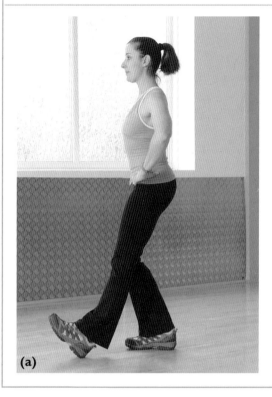

(a)

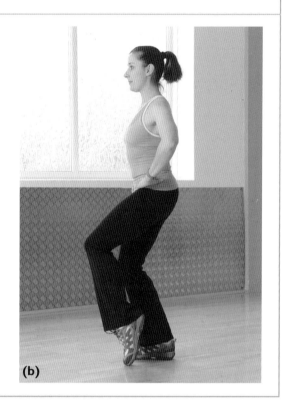

(b)

Heel toe

Purpose: to mobilise the ankles.

Preparation

Stand in correct upright posture, with hands on hips.

Action

Gently draw in the abdomen and transfer the weight onto one leg. Keeping the supporting knee soft, alternately flex and point the other foot (heel/toe) to the floor. Repeat as required before changing feet.

Technique tips

- Ensure that the action comes from the ankle and not the knee.
- Pull up out of the supporting hip to avoid pushing out to the side.
- Keep the supporting knee soft and correctly aligned.
- Keep the spine long and the chest open.
- Keep the movement slow and controlled.

Figure 8.7 Foot mobility

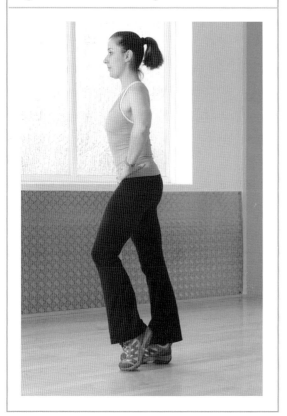

Foot mobility

Purpose: to mobilise stiff ankles and feet and promote circulation.

Preparation

Stand in correct upright posture, with feet together and hands on hips. Lift the heel of the right foot off the floor, keeping the base of the toe joints pressed down. Keep the hips level and knees soft.

Action

Gently draw in the abdomen as the weight is transferred through alternate feet lifting the arch of the foot as high as possible. Maintain an upright stance throughout. Lift through the supporting hip to avoid rocking, and keep the spine long.

Technique tips

* Keep knee aligned over foot.
* Ensure that all toes are weight bearing – watch out for big and little toes coming off the floor.
* Hinge at the toe joints and emphasise the lift through the arches.
* Avoid rocking the hips from side to side – the action is in the feet.
* Maintain a lifted posture.
* Keep the movements slow and controlled.

Figure 8.8 Warm-up squat

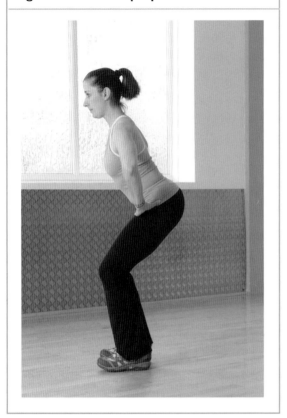

Action

Gently draw in the abdomen and bend the knees, hinging at the hips and lowering the buttocks a short distance. Return to upright standing position. Repeat as required.

Technique tips

- Keep the spine long and buttocks relaxed.
- Ensure that knees are tracking in line with the feet.
- Tighten the buttocks to return to the upright standing position.
- Fully extend knees and hips on return.
- Be sure to relax the buttocks before repeating the bend.
- Do not bend too low.

Warm-up squat

Purpose: to mobilise the knees and hips.

Preparation

Stand in correct upright posture, with hands on hips.

Figure 8.9 Knee bend

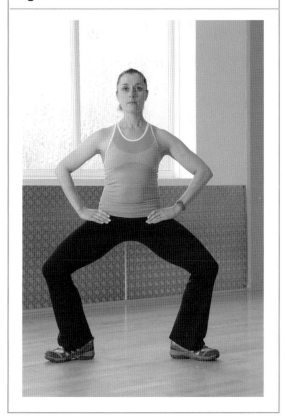

Action

Gently draw in the abdomen and bend the knees, keeping the heels down and knees aligned with toes. Keep the spine lifted and the head up. Slowly straighten the knees, taking care not to lock them out. Repeat as required.

Technique tips

* Maintain upright posture – avoid moving the buttocks backwards.
* Ensure that knees move outwards and in line with toes.
* Visualise the tailbone moving towards the floor.
* Keep the bend shallow – avoid bending below 90 degrees.
* Vary the muscular focus as the knees straighten – (a) by drawing the quadriceps up and (b) by drawing the adductors up.

Caution: Reduce the depth of the bend if this pulls on the adductors.

Knee bend

Purpose: to mobilise the knees and hips.

Preparation

Stand in correct upright posture, with feet wider than hips, comfortably turned out. Place hands on hips. This is a wider stance than the warm-up squat.

Figure 8.10 Knee raise

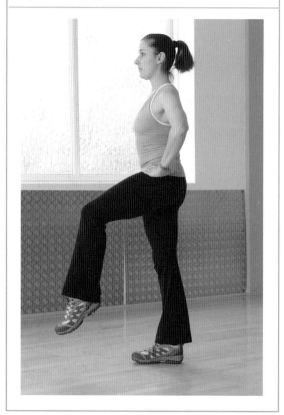

Action

Gently draw in the abdomen and lift alternate knees up in front to a comfortable height, keeping the back lifted. Avoid dropping into the supporting hip during the transition. Repeat as required.

Technique tips

- Lengthen the torso and lift out of the hips.
- Replace the foot directly under the hip to prevent the pelvis rocking from side to side.
- Keep the chest lifted throughout and avoid dipping towards the knee.
- Add upper body rotation by touching hand to opposite knee.

Knee raise

Purpose: to mobilise the knees and hips.

Preparation

Stand in correct upright posture, hands on hips.

Figure 8.11 Trunk curl

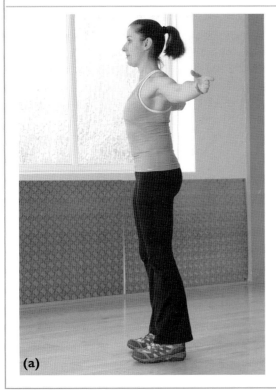
(a)

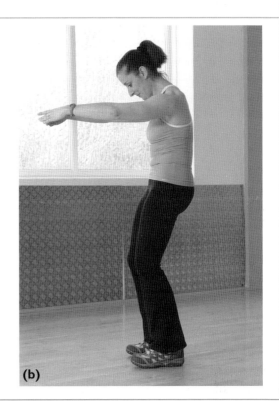
(b)

Trunk curl

Purpose: to open the chest and loosen the upper body.

Preparation

Stand in correct upright posture, with arms out to the side at shoulder height.

Action

Gently draw in the abdominals and tilt the pelvis, curling the tailbone under and rounding the upper body forwards. Allow the arms to curl forwards with the back. Return to the upright standing position, lengthening the spine and opening the arms to the sides. Repeat as required.

Technique tips

- Relax the head forwards during the trunk curl.
- Draw the shoulder blades down as the trunk curls forwards and keep the neck long.
- Lift out of the hips and lengthen as you open.
- Feel the chest lengthening as the arms reach to the sides.
- Avoid pushing the chest forwards on the extension.
- Keep the movement slow and continuous.

Figure 8.12 Arm circle

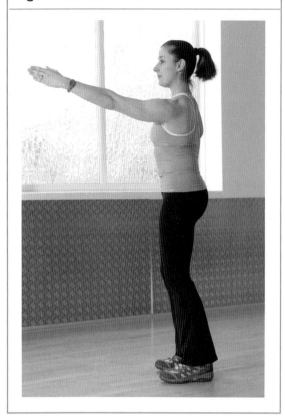

Action

Gently draw in the abdomen and take one arm around in a slow circle, keeping the hips and shoulders facing forwards. Make the circle as large as possible. Repeat as required before changing to the other side.

Technique tips

* Keep the arm close to the body throughout.
* Begin with a small range of movement and gradually increase with each repetition.
* Emphasise the full circular movement, paying particular attention to the backward phase.
* Avoid arching the back as the arm moves behind.
* Keep hips and shoulders facing forwards as the arm circles behind.
* Keep the movement slow and continuous.

Arm circle

Purpose: to mobilise the shoulder and open the chest.

Preparation

Stand in correct upright posture, with arms relaxed by sides.

Figure 8.13 Neck mobility

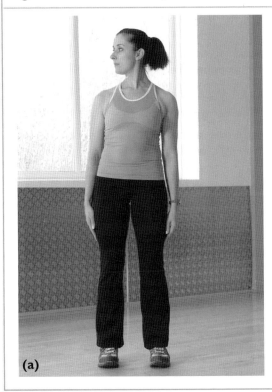

(a)

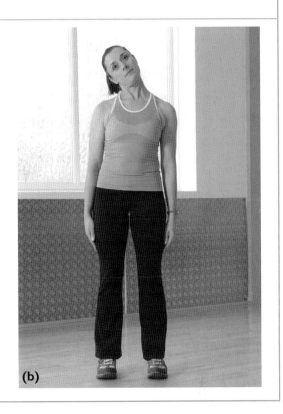

(b)

Neck mobility

Purpose: to release tension in the neck.

Preparation

Stand in correct upright posture, with arms relaxed by sides.

Action

(a) Gently draw in the abdomen and, keeping the shoulders relaxed, slowly turn the head to look over one shoulder, pause and return to the centre, keeping the neck long. Repeat on the other side.

(b) Gently draw in the abdomen and tilt the head sideways, taking the ear towards the shoulder. Repeat on the other side.

Technique tips

- Keep shoulder blades sliding down and chest lifted.
- Avoid tipping to the side as the head moves.
- Lengthen the spine each time on recovery.
- Keep the movements slow and controlled.

DYNAMIC STRETCHES

Static v dynamic stretching in the warm-up

Static stretches are not recommended as part of the warm-up. It is more beneficial to lengthen the muscles dynamically than hold them in a static position. Not only does this prepare for the activity in a more functional way but it also continues to warm and loosen the joints, which may be feeling quite restricted and stiff following childbirth. Dynamic stretching should not be confused with ballistic stretching, which takes the joint beyond its normal range of movement using momentum; dynamic stretching keeps movements within the normal range of the joint but is movement specific. Static stretching has its place at the end of the session.

How do you perform dynamic stretches?

Examples of dynamic stretches are hamstrings curls to lengthen the quadriceps; knee lifts to lengthen the gluteals (and possibly hamstrings); pelvic tilts to lengthen the hip flexors; and trunk curls to lengthen the pectorals.

EXERCISES FOR MUSCULAR STRENGTH AND ENDURANCE

Important!

Breathing should focus on exhaling with recruitment of TrA to ensure that the local stabilisers are working together as a group. As before, both should be cued for the first repetition and normal breathing encouraged throughout. It is not necessary to give constant reminders to activate TrA – once they have been recruited they should continue to work for the duration of the exercise.

Figure 8.16 Forward lunge

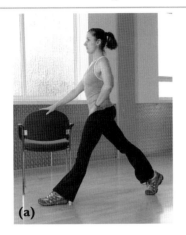 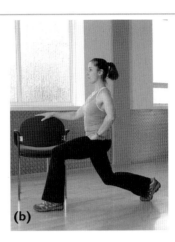

(a) (b)

Standing exercises

Forward lunge

Purpose: to strengthen the gluteals and quadriceps and train good technique for kneeling down to the floor.

Preparation

Stand in correct upright posture, sideways to a support and holding on with one hand if needed, other hand on hip. Take a large step back with one foot into a split stance, maintaining hip width, and lift the back heel off the floor. Centre the weight between the legs and lengthen the spine.

Action

Inhale to prepare then, when exhaling, recruit TrA and bend both knees, lowering the back knee towards the floor. Keep the body weight centred to ensure correct knee/ankle alignment. Return to standing, keeping the spine lifted and long and the shoulders down. Repeat as required before changing legs. Maintain natural breathing.

Technique tips

- Maintain correct postural alignment throughout.
- Keep the front knee aligned over the ankle and back knee under the hip.
- Avoid locking out the knee on return to standing.
- Lengthen the spine away from the floor as the knees bend.
- Slide the shoulder blades and ribcage down.
- Look straight ahead – avoid looking down.
- Perform slowly and with control.
- Keep the range of movement small initially and progress to a deeper bend when strength has been gained.

Caution: Stop and check alignment if pain or discomfort is felt in the pelvis or the knees. This is an intensive exercise and should commence with low repetitions. Women recovering from PGP may find this exercise uncomfortable.

Progression

Once strength has been gained, this exercise can be performed holding weights.

Figure 8.17 Curtsey lunge

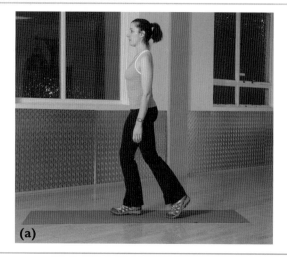

(a)

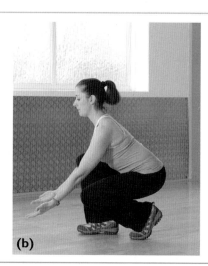

(b)

Curtsey lunge

Purpose: To strengthen the gluteals and quadriceps and train correct bending and lifting technique.

Preparation

Stand in correct upright posture, with a shortened split stance, maintaining hip width. This should be a natural stance used for picking something up.

Action

Inhale to prepare and when exhaling recruit TrA; lift the back heel off the floor and bend both knees, hinging forwards from the hips. Lower the buttocks towards the heel of the back foot, the arms reaching to the floor in front – as if to pick something up. Tighten the gluteals and drive up to upright standing position using the buttocks, drawing the arms back in towards the body. Repeat as required before changing legs. Maintain natural breathing.

Technique tips

- Ensure that the knees and hips flex at the same time.
- Keep the spine in neutral as it hinges forwards from the hips.
- Keep the body weight slightly forward.
- Avoid lifting the shoulders when bending.
- Drive up through the gluteals, extending knees and hips together.
- Return to upright standing position each time.
- Ensure that the arms come back in towards the body for the lifting phase.
- Slide the shoulder blades and ribcage down during the lifting phase.

Note: P239 shows how this exercise is used for bending and lifting baby. Whilst baby should not be used during the exercise it is important to practice bringing the arms in on the upward phase so it becomes automatic when baby is involved.

Figure 8.18 Squat

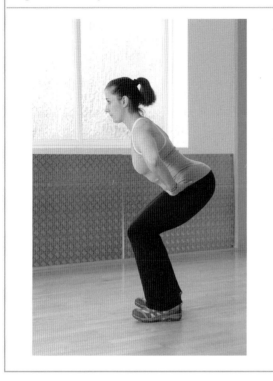

Squat

Purpose: to strengthen the gluteals, quadriceps and hamstrings and improve posture.

Preparation

Stand in correct upright posture with hands on hips. Take a slightly wider stance if needed to maintain a stable base and good joint alignment.

Action

Inhale to prepare and when exhaling recruit TrA; bend the knees and hinge at the hips, lowering the buttocks towards the floor (not lower than 90 degrees). Tighten the gluteals and drive up to upright standing position using the buttocks. Repeat as required. Maintain natural breathing.

Technique tips

- Ensure that knees are tracking in line with the feet.
- Do not allow knees to go beyond the toes.
- Ensure that body flexes forwards from the hips as buttocks push backwards, to maintain balance over the feet.
- Maintain rib–hip connection.
- Extend knees and hips together.
- Tight calves may reduce the range of movement.
- Draw shoulder blades and ribcage down.

Caution: Reduce the range of movement if discomfort is felt in the knees.

Figure 8.19 Squat with balance

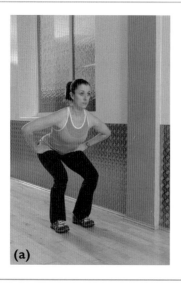

(a)

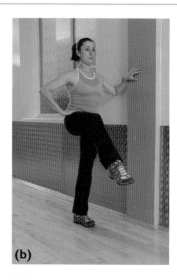

(b)

Squat with balance

Purpose: To strengthen the gluteals, quadriceps and hamstrings and to improve stability, balance and proprioception.

Preparation

As for squat above.

Action

Inhale to prepare. When exhaling recruit TrA and squat down as before but on the upward phase lift one knee, pulling up on the supporting side to prevent the hip dropping. Lower the foot slowly to the floor on the next squat. Repeat moving from two feet to one alternately. Maintain natural breathing.

Technique tips

As for squat, plus:
- Transfer the weight onto one leg at the beginning of the upward phase.
- Lift up through the supporting side to keep the hips level.
- Pause for a split second at the top of the move.

Caution: Women recovering from PGP may find this exercise uncomfortable.

Progression

One leg squat – as above but standing next to a support, remain with one knee lifted and squat on one leg. Progress to unsupported standing.

Figure 8.20 Calf raise

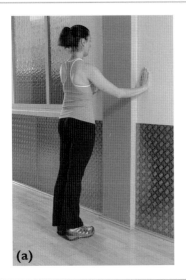

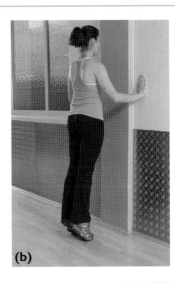

(a)

(b)

Calf raise

Purpose: to strengthen gastrocnemius and improve circulation. This exercise may also be helpful for PFM recruitment.

Preparation

Stand in correct upright posture, facing a wall. Step back one pace from the support, resting the hands at shoulder height and look straight ahead. Centre the weight over the feet and soften the knees.

Action

Inhale to prepare and as you exhale recruit TrA and slowly rise up onto the toes, keeping feet facing forwards and weight spread evenly on both feet. Lift the arches of the feet and lengthen the spine. Slowly lower the heels to touch lightly on the floor, keeping the weight slightly forward. Repeat as required. Maintain natural breathing.

Technique tips

- Keep the ankles lifted to avoid rolling the foot inwards or outwards.
- Keep the weight spread across the base of all toe joints.
- Lift the arches of the feet as high as possible.
- Avoid rolling back onto the heels when lowering.
- Maintain correct spinal alignment throughout – avoid body sway.
- Slide the shoulder blades down.
- Perform slowly and with control.

NB: Combining with a PFME may be helpful for women who are having difficulty recruiting these muscles. Encourage PFME as the heels lift, and hold the two contractions for a few seconds before lowering both heels with control. A faster action can be used to activate the fast-twitch fibres of PFM, ensuring that the lowering phase is still controlled.

Figure 8.21 Standing gluteal raise

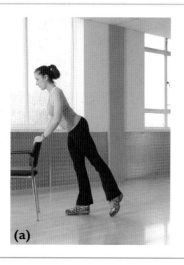

(a)

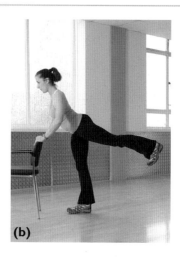

(b)

Standing gluteal raise

Purpose: to strengthen gluteus maximus to aid pelvic stability, improve posture and assist with bending and lifting movements.

Preparation

Stand in correct upright posture, two paces away from a wall or high-backed chair, facing the support. Lean into the support, hinging at the hips, and place hands on the chair or wall (at chest height with fingers facing upwards if at the wall). Lift through the supporting hip and transfer the weight onto one leg. Extend the other leg on the floor behind and lengthen from the hip.

Action

Inhale to prepare and as you exhale recruit TrA, squeeze the buttocks and slowly lift the leg up and back. Keep the upper body forward with both hips square to the wall. Lower the leg to the floor, keeping the hips level and upper body still. Repeat as required before changing legs. Maintain natural breathing.

Technique tips

- Activating the gluteals prior to lifting will assist muscle recruitment.
- The upper body should remain tilted forwards from the hips throughout.
- Keep the hips over the feet.
- Keep lifted on the supporting side – fatigue will cause the hip to push out to the side.
- Keep supporting knee soft.
- Slide the shoulder blades and ribcage down.
- Only lift the leg as high as correct hip alignment allows.
- Perform slowly and with control.

Caution: Slow, controlled movements are essential for this exercise to avoid stress to the lower back. Avoid lifting the leg too high as this will cause the back to arch. Women recovering from PGP may find this exercise uncomfortable.

Alternative

This exercise can also be performed on the floor (*see* page 122).

Figure 8.22 Inner range training for gluteus maximus

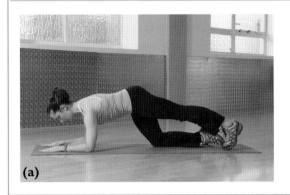
(a)

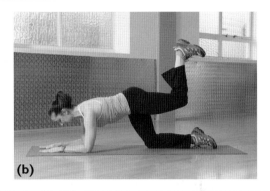
(b)

Inner range training for gluteus maximus

Purpose: To shorten stretch-weakened gluteus maximus and increase strength in the inner range.

This is more effective in a kneeling position but can also be done standing. Preparation and action are as for gluteal raise above, but with the knee bent to 90 degrees. This reduces the input from the hamstrings and concentrates the workload on gluteus maximus. Perform a few repetitions with the knee bent, checking all technique tips as above, particularly hip and spinal alignment. Hold in the lifted position for a few seconds, maintaining alignment and then lower. Maintain natural breathing.

Progress this by increasing the length of hold of the raised leg, which must be at full hip extension to work the inner range effectively. Work towards holding for 10 seconds and repeat 10 times.

Caution: Loss of correct spinal alignment can easily occur with the knee bent – close observation is essential to ensure that the lower back is not compromised.

Figure 8.23 Wall press-up

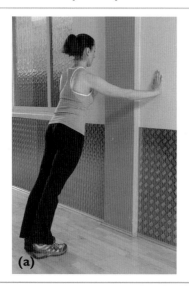

(a)

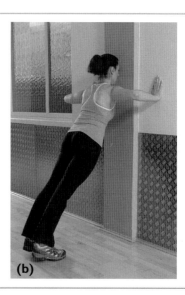

(b)

Wall press-up

Purpose: to strengthen the pectorals and triceps to assist with lifting and carrying.

Preparation

Stand in correct upright posture, facing a wall. Step back two paces from the wall, lean forwards from the feet and position hands on the wall at shoulder height but wider than shoulders. Ensure that fingers are pointing upwards and elbows are soft.

Action

Inhale to prepare and as you exhale recruit TrA, bend the elbows, and lower the upper body towards the wall, keeping the spine in neutral. Allow the heels to lift if necessary. Ensure that the elbows bend in line with the wrists. Slowly straighten the arms and return to the starting position. Repeat as required. Maintain natural breathing.

Technique tips

- Maintain correct head alignment.
- Slide shoulder blades down and lengthen the spine.
- Ensure that elbows bend over the wrists – if not, take the hands wider.
- Avoid locking out the elbows on the extension.
- Keep the movement slow, smooth and controlled.

Alternative

This exercise can also be performed on the floor (*see* page 119).

Figure 8.24 Seated leg extension

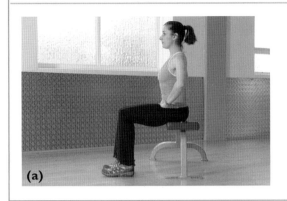 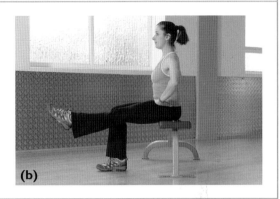

(a) (b)

Seated exercises

Seated leg extension

Purpose: to strengthen vastus medialis (medial quadriceps), to increase knee stability and rebalance quadriceps group strength.

Preparation

Sit in correct upright posture towards the front of an upright chair, with hands on hips.

Action

Inhale to prepare and as you exhale recruit TrA and slowly straighten one knee, keeping the top of the thigh on the chair. Focus on the final full extension of the knee without locking out. Lift up out of the hips and keep the spine lengthened. Repeat as required before changing legs. Maintain natural breathing.

Technique tips

- Maintain upright posture throughout.
- Create a strong, resisted feeling as you straighten the knee.
- Avoid leaning back as the leg straightens.
- Slide shoulder blades and ribcage down.
- Perform the exercise slowly and with control.

> **Figure 8.25 Bridge with heel raise**
>
>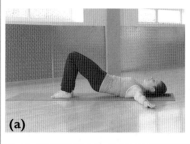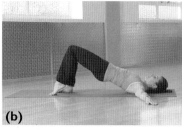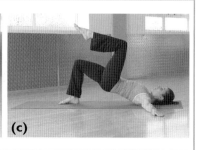
>
> (a)   (b)   (c)

Floor exercises

Getting down to the floor

Recruit TrA before bending the knees and use the large muscles in the legs to lower one knee to the floor. Bring the other knee down and move onto hands and knees. Sit the body down to one side and turn around into a seated position keeping knees and feet aligned.

Bridge with heel raise

Purpose: to strengthen the gluteus maximus, medius and minimus for improved posture and pelvic stability.

Preparation

Perform the first part of the spine curl as detailed on page 48.

Action

Hold in the lifted position and transfer the weight onto one side. Tighten the gluteals and lift the opposite heel off the floor, keeping the hips level. Lower the heel without dropping the hip and repeat on the other side. Lower the hips to the floor, maintaining neutral.

Technique tips

- Tighten the buttocks prior to lifting, to activate gluteus maximus.
- Poor use of gluteals will induce hamstring cramps – lower hips carefully to the floor if this occurs.
- Keep the buttocks lifted but avoid over-squeezing.
- Do not allow the hips to move.
- Draw the ribcage down.
- Keep the spine long.

Progression

Lift the knee up over the hip, keeping the pelvis level and hold for a few seconds, maintaining good alignment.

Caution: Women recovering from PGP may find this exercise uncomfortable.

Alternative

Hold in the lifted bridge position, with both feet on the floor and perform scissor arms or arm circles (*see* pages 33 and 35). Increasing the length of hold builds up gluteal strength.

Figure 8.26 Press-up

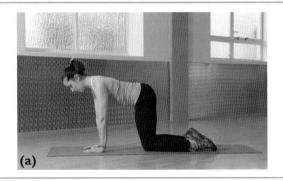

(a)

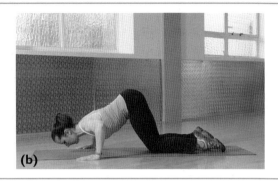

(b)

Press-up

Purpose: to strengthen the pectorals and triceps to assist with lifting, carrying and everyday activities.

Preparation

Go down onto hands and knees in correct postural alignment (*see* page 31), hands wider than shoulders and fingers facing forwards. Slide the shoulders down and soften the elbows. Move the body weight forwards onto your hands, keeping the head correctly aligned.

Action

Inhale to prepare and as you exhale recruit TrA and bend the elbows, slowly lowering the upper body towards the floor, aligning elbows over wrists. Keep the weight forwards as you slowly push up to the starting position, taking care not to lock out the elbows. Repeat as required. Maintain natural breathing.

Technique tips

- Keep the head aligned with spine – do not allow the forehead to drop.
- Aim to touch the nose on the floor between the hands.
- Ensure that elbows are over wrists when bending – stop and take the hands wider if necessary.

- Ensure that the elbows fully extend but do not lock out.
- Maintain correct spinal alignment throughout.
- Keep the movement slow, smooth and controlled.

Progression

1 When 20 press-ups can comfortably be performed in this position, keep the hands where they are but move the body weight further forwards and repeat with head in front of hands.
2 Move the hands and body weight further forwards.

Alternatives

1 If this position is uncomfortable for the knees or wrists, or tingling/numbness is experienced in the fingers, try this exercise standing at the wall (*see* page 116).
2 Alternatively, placing a small rolled towel under the heel of the hand may be enough to prevent these symptoms occurring in the wrists and fingers.
3 If wrist alignment is a problem for both exercises, perform the chest flye described on page 34 and increase the resistance by holding small hand weights.

Figure 8.27 Threading through

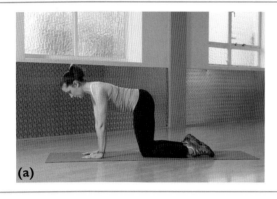

(a)

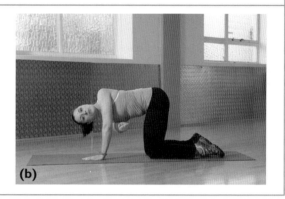

(b)

Threading through

Purpose: To mobilise the thoracic spine and reduce stiffness.

Preparation

Go down onto hands and knees in correct postural alignment for four point kneeling (*see* page 31).

Action

Inhale to prepare and as you exhale recruit TrA and transfer your weight onto your left arm without sinking into the shoulder. With your right arm, reach under your torso and out to the left side, rotating from the middle of the back upwards. Return to starting position and repeat on the other side. Maintain natural breathing.

Technique tips

- Lengthen the spine.
- Keep the supporting elbow soft and lift out of the shoulder.
- Draw the shoulder blades down your back.
- Keep the weight evenly distributed on both knees.

- Avoid twisting in the pelvis.
- Keep the head aligned with the spine and rotate from the middle of the back.
- Reach the arm as far away as possible.
- Pause and try to reach a little further.

Progression

Instead of replacing the hand on the floor, lift the arm out to the side and sweep upwards until the fingers are pointing towards the ceiling. Move the head with the spine to finish looking up at the hand. This movement rotates the torso in the opposite direction and opens the chest. Keep the supporting elbow soft and shoulder blades drawn down. Do not allow the pelvis to move – the rotation is all in the thoracic spine. This exercise becomes quite demanding on the supporting arm.

Figure 8.28 Thoracic extension

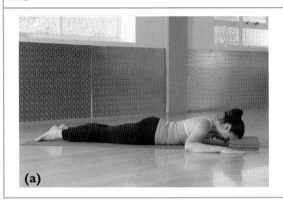

(a)

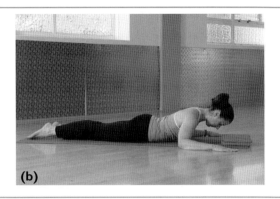

(b)

Thoracic extension

Purpose: to strengthen lower trapezius to improve kyphotic posture and increase spinal mobility.

Preparation

Lie prone (breast comfort permitting), with arms on the floor to the sides at shoulder level, elbows bent to 90 degrees and forearms on the floor. Relax head forwards on the floor or a cushion. Bring legs together in neutral position, lengthened from the hip.

Action

Inhale to prepare and while exhaling recruit TrA and, using the forearms for support, lift the lower ribcage off the floor. Lengthen the spine forwards while lifting and slide the shoulder blades down. Pause, continuing to breathe before lowering, lengthening the torso away from the hips. Keep the repetitions low. Maintain natural breathing.

Technique tips

- Lift from the lower ribcage.
- Keep the head aligned in neutral – do not drop it back or push the chin forwards.
- Extend the spine rather than curling it back.
- Lengthen the tailbone towards the feet.
- Avoid any movement in the pelvis or lower back.
- Placing a small rolled towel under the abdomen may help maintain pelvic alignment.

Caution: This is not a backbend! Allowing the abdomen to collapse into the floor will increase the pressure on the lower back.

Figure 8.29 Kneeling gluteal raise

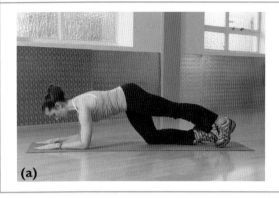

(a)

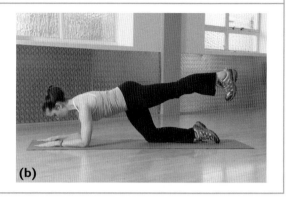

(b)

Kneeling gluteal raise

Purpose: to strengthen gluteus maximus to aid pelvic stability, improve posture and assist with bending and lifting movements.

Preparation

Go down onto elbows and knees, keeping spine in correct alignment, with elbows under shoulders and forearms facing forwards. Straighten the right leg behind with foot flexed, toes resting on the floor, keeping hips level and square to the floor.

Action

Inhale to prepare and as you exhale recruit TrA, tighten the buttocks and slowly lift the leg, keeping the hips level and square to the floor. Lower to the floor, lengthening the leg away from the hip and keeping the hips and upper body still. Repeat as required before changing legs. Maintain natural breathing.

Technique tips

- Activate the gluteals prior to lifting, to assist correct muscle recruitment.
- Lengthen the leg away from the hip, but avoid locking out the knee.
- Lift through the supporting hip to avoid rolling over on the knee.

- Keep both hip bones facing the floor.
- Slide the shoulder blades down.
- Only lift the leg as high as correct hip alignment allows.
- Perform slowly and with control.

Caution: Lifting the leg too high will cause the back to arch. Women recovering from PGP may find this exercise uncomfortable.

Alternative

If this position is uncomfortable for knees or breasts, try the standing version (*see* page 114).

Inner range training for gluteus maximus

Purpose: To shorten stretch-weakened gluteus maximus and increase strength in the inner range.

Preparation and action are as for the kneeling glute raise above, but with knee bent to 90 degrees. This reduces the input from the hamstrings and concentrates the workload on the gluteus maximus. Perform a few repetitions with knee bent, checking all technique tips as above, particularly hip and spinal alignment. Hold in the lifted position for a few seconds, maintaining alignment, and then lower. Maintain natural breathing.

Progress this by increasing the length of hold

Figure 8.30 Outer thigh raise

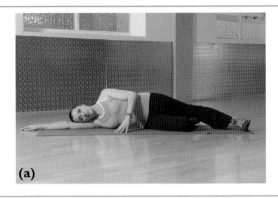

(a)

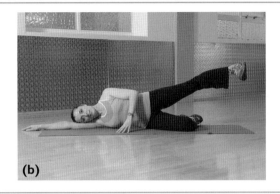

(b)

of the raised leg, which must be in full hip extension to effectively work inner range. Work towards holding for 10 seconds. Repeat as required.

Caution: Loss of correct spinal alignment can easily occur with the knee bent – close observation is essential to ensure that the lower back is not compromised.

Adaptation

If this is difficult to hold, instructors can assist by supporting the knee at the appropriate height. They can then ask the client to hold the leg without dropping and/or help the client to control the lowering from this height.

Outer thigh raise

Purpose: to strengthen the gluteus medius and minimus muscles to aid pelvic stability.

Preparation

Lie on the side in correct spinal alignment (*see* page 30), with underneath leg bent, knee slightly forward and top leg straight in line with the body. Rest head on the underneath arm and lift the waistband away from the floor. Flex the top foot and rotate the leg forwards so the side of the thigh faces the ceiling and the toes are angled downwards. Lean slightly forwards onto the top arm, which is resting on the floor.

Action

Inhale to prepare and as you exhale recruit TrA and slowly lift the top leg, keeping the hip rotated forwards and the knee soft. Lift as high as the joint permits, keeping the hips stacked and not sinking into the underneath waistband. Lower slowly with control without resting the foot on the floor. Repeat as required before changing legs. Maintain natural breathing.

Technique tips

- Lengthen the leg away from the hip.
- Avoid dipping into the floor at the waist as the leg lifts.
- Maintain correct spinal alignment throughout.
- Create a feeling of resistance in the leg as it lowers.
- Bend the top knee if it feels uncomfortable.
- Avoid overflexing the foot and creating tension in the lower leg.
- Keep the hip rotated forwards – allowing it to drop back will involve the quadriceps and hip flexors, rather than the intended muscles.
- Keep the top shoulder drawn down.
- Perform slowly and carefully – don't be tempted to throw the leg up.

Caution: Women recovering from PGP may find this exercise uncomfortable.

Figure 8.31 Side lying knee raise

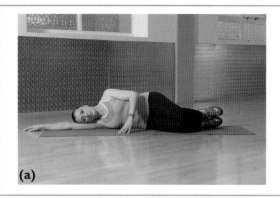

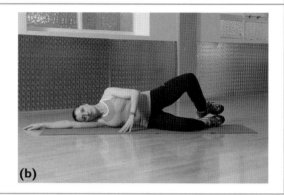

(a)　　　　　(b)

Side lying knee raise

Purpose: to strengthen gluteus medius to assist with pelvic stability.

Preparation

Lie on the side in correct alignment, with knees and feet together and knees bent to 45 degrees. Extend the underneath arm beneath head, top arm relaxed on the floor in front, with shoulder drawn down.

Action

Inhale to prepare and while exhaling recruit TrA and lift the top knee, keeping feet together and rotating at the hip. Do not allow the pelvis to rock backwards. Lower with control and repeat as required.

Technique tips

- Maintain correct spinal alignment.
- Keep the hips vertically stacked throughout.
- Lift only as far as correct pelvic alignment can be maintained.
- Avoid rolling back onto the buttocks.
- Feel the buttock muscles drawing the leg around.
- Keep the top shoulder drawn down and spine long.

Caution: Women recovering from PGP may find this exercise uncomfortable.

Figure 8.32 Inner thigh raise

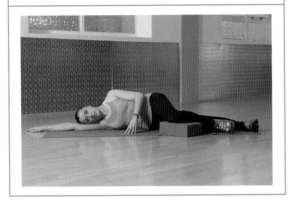

Inner thigh raise

Purpose: to strengthen the adductors to aid pelvic stability.

Preparation

Lie on the side in correct alignment, with head resting on the underneath arm. Bring the top leg forwards, bend the knee and place a couple of cushions underneath the knee to maintain knee/hip alignment. Straighten the underneath leg and ensure that the inner thigh faces upwards. Rest the top hand on the floor in front for support, with shoulder relaxed down. Lengthen the spine and lift the waistband away from the floor.

Action

Inhale to prepare and as you exhale recruit TrA and lift the underneath leg towards the ceiling, keeping the inner thigh uppermost and the knee soft. Lower with control, keeping the upper body relaxed on the floor. Repeat as required before changing legs.

Technique tips

- Maintain correct alignment throughout.
- Lengthen the leg away from the hip.
- Avoid sinking into the underneath waistband as the leg lifts.
- Soften the knee more if discomfort is felt in the knee joint.
- Avoid overflexing the foot and creating tension in the lower leg.
- Move the top knee down towards the feet if discomfort is felt in the buttocks.
- Perform the exercise slowly and with control.

Caution: Women recovering from PGP may find this exercise uncomfortable.

Figure 8.37 Rainbow stretch

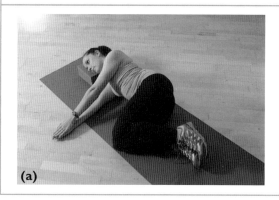

(a)

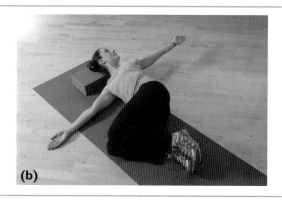

(b)

Rainbow stretch

Purpose: to mobilise the thoracic spine and stretch the pectorals.

Preparation

Lie on the side in correct alignment, with a pillow or block under the head to maintain spinal alignment. Bend both knees up in front and extend the arms on the floor in front at chest height with palms together and shoulders relaxed.

Action

Gently draw in the abdomen and lift the top arm up to the ceiling, keeping the shoulder drawn down and turning the head to look upwards. Continue the movement over to the other side, following with the head. Pause with both arms open to the side just below shoulder height and hips stacked, continuing to breathe. To return, use the abdominal muscles to draw the body back to side lying, reaching the arm up and over the chest in a straight line to return to starting position. Maintain natural breathing.

Technique tips

- Movement is limited by thoracic mobility – rolling onto the buttocks will allow the rotation to occur through the pelvis and lumbar spine, which defeats the object of the exercise.
- Ensure that pelvis and lumbar spine remain still – avoid rolling back.
- Keep the hips stacked throughout.
- Lengthen the arm away from the shoulder.
- Draw the shoulder blades down.
- Release the neck as it turns.
- Pause and release in an open chest stretch.
- Initiate the return with the abdominals by drawing ribs across to opposite hips.
- Keep the movement slow and controlled.

SEATED STRETCHES

Maintaining correct posture when seated

During seated stretches a block or cushion can be placed under the sit bones to assist the maintenance of correct upright posture.

Seated hamstring stretch

Purpose: to lengthen the hamstrings.

Preparation

Sit on the floor in correct upright posture, with one leg straight out in front, knee soft, and the other leg bent to the side in a comfortable position. Lift up onto the sit bones and support hands on the floor behind.

Action

Gently draw in the abdomen and press down onto the hands to lengthen the spine. Slowly incline the body forwards until you feel a stretch in the back of the straight leg. Keep the knees and toes of the straight leg facing up. Repeat on the other leg. Maintain natural breathing.

Technique tips

- Maintain lengthened spine – do not roll back off the sit bones.
- Keep the chest lifted to encourage length.
- Keep the knee soft on the stretching leg.
- If no stretch is experienced, push down on the hands and lift the buttocks slightly back, keeping the heel in place. Be sure to move both buttocks back together – this lengthens the hamstrings further.
- If correct alignment can be maintained, place the hands on the floor in front.
- Move into position slowly.

Figure 8.39 Seated gluteal stretch

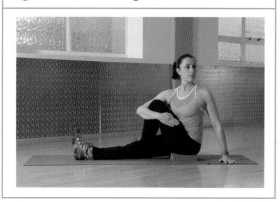

Seated gluteal stretch

Purpose: to lengthen the gluteals and increase thoracic mobility.

Preparation

Seated on the floor in correct upright posture, with right leg straight out in front, knee soft. Bend the left leg over the right and place the foot flat on the floor, close to the right leg. Lift up onto your sit bones and support your hands on the floor behind.

Action

Gently draw in the abdomen and wrap the right arm around the left knee, gently hugging the knee towards the chest. Lengthen the spine and gently rotate the upper body around to the left keeping both buttocks firmly on the floor. Feel a stretch in the left buttock and right torso. Repeat on the other leg. Maintain natural breathing.

Technique tips

- Cradle the knee into chest with the elbow and forearm.
- Lengthen the spine away from sit bones.
- Slide the shoulder blades down.
- Move the foot closer to hip if the stretch is not felt.
- Keep both buttocks firmly on the floor.
- Avoid the rotation if breasts are uncomfortable, or perform lying supine (*see* page 128).
- Breathe throughout.

Progression

Pause in rotation and lift up out of the sit bones. Slowly rotate a little further.

Seated adductor stretch

Purpose: to lengthen the adductors.

Preparation

Sit on the floor in correct upright posture, with soles of the feet together and knees open to the side. Lift up onto sit bones and support with hands on the floor behind.

Action

Gently draw in the abdomen and, using the arms behind for support, slide the buttocks in towards the heels until a stretch is felt in the inner thighs. Relax the knees. Maintain natural breathing.

Technique tips

- Push the body weight slightly forwards with the hands.
- Avoid locking out the elbows.
- Lengthen the spine away from sit bones.
- Keep both buttocks firmly on the floor.
- Place hands on the floor in front if this is more comfortable.
- Do not attempt to push too far with this stretch.

Caution: Women recovering from PGP may need reassurance to stretch the adductors as they may feel quite anxious about this area (*see* page 76). It is vital that they move into this stretch slowly to allow the muscles time to adapt – moving quickly and/or forcefully into position, without the necessary care and attention, will cause pain!

Figure 8.41   Seated pectoral stretch

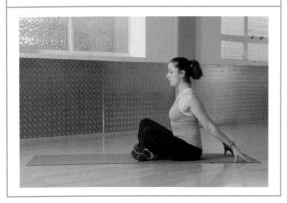

Seated pectoral stretch

Purpose: to lengthen the pectorals and improve posture.

Preparation

Sit on the floor in correct upright posture, with legs in a comfortable position. Without taking the weight backwards, rest the fingertips on the floor behind the buttocks.

Action

Gently draw in the abdomen, lengthen the spine and open the chest drawing the elbows back. Draw the ribcage down to prevent the chest lifting and maintain correct spinal alignment. Feel a stretch across the chest and the front of the shoulders. Maintain natural breathing.

Technique tips

* Keep the weight on the buttocks and avoid leaning back onto the arms.
* Lengthen the spine away from sit bones.
* Open the chest but do not lift it.
* Draw the ribcage and shoulder blades down.
* Avoid locking out the elbows.

Figure 8.42 Seated trapezius stretch

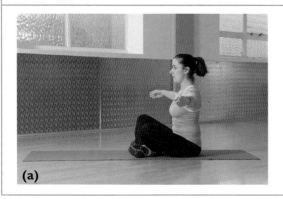
(a)

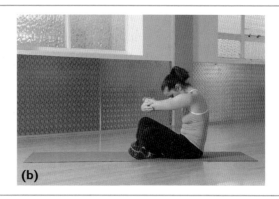
(b)

Seated trapezius stretch

Purpose: to reduce tension in mid-trapezius muscles as a result of postural changes.

Preparation

Sit on the floor in correct upright posture, with legs in a comfortable position. Extend the arms to the sides at shoulder height and draw the shoulder blades down.

Action

Gently draw in the abdomen, tilt the pelvis (pubic bone up) and draw the arms forwards in front of the chest, curving the spine, including the head. Bend the elbows and take hold of the opposite forearm and press the shoulders forwards. Feel a stretch between the shoulder blades. Maintain natural breathing.

Technique tips

- Draw the shoulder blades down and keep the neck long.
- Avoid sinking into the floor on the pelvic tilt.
- Lengthen the tailbone under but keep the spine long.
- Keep the elbows bent in front.
- Keep shoulders over hips – avoid leaning forwards from the hips.
- Allow the head to complete the spine curl.

Figure 8.47 Standing gastrocnemius stretch

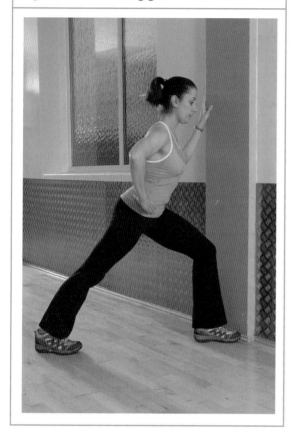

Action

Gently draw in the abdomen and bend the front knee, pressing the back heel into the floor with the knee straight. Keep both hips facing forwards. Repeat using the other leg. Maintain natural breathing.

Technique tips

- Lean slightly forwards with the upper body to maintain a diagonal line from head to heel.
- Keep the chest lifted and open.
- Slide the shoulder blades down.
- Keep the front knee aligned over ankle.
- Feel the stretch in the bulky part of the calf.
- Move the foot further back for a more intensive stretch.
- Use the wall or a chair for support if required.

Adaptation

If the stretch cannot be felt, stand on the bottom stair and hang the heel of one foot off the edge. Bend the supporting knee and allow the heel to drop. Avoid locking out the knee of the stretching leg.

Standing gastrocnemius stretch

Purpose: to lengthen and reduce tension in the gastrocnemius and assist postural correction.

Preparation

Stand in correct upright posture, with hands on hips. Keeping the feet hip-width apart, take a large step backwards with the left foot, keeping both heels down and the feet facing forwards.

Figure 8.48 Standing soleus stretch

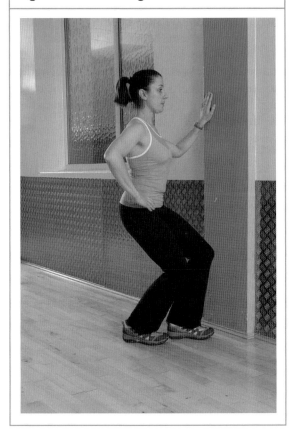

Action

Gently draw in the abdomen and bend both knees, keeping the back heel on the floor. Move the weight towards the back foot but maintain correct spinal alignment. Feel a stretch in the lower calf. Repeat on the other leg. Maintain natural breathing throughout.

Technique tips

- Keep the chest lifted and open.
- Slide the shoulder blades down.
- Lift up out of the hips and keep them level.
- Maintain correct alignment in both knees.
- Adjust the body weight towards the back foot if the stretch is not felt.
- Do not allow the back to arch.
- Use the wall or a chair for support if required.

Standing soleus stretch

Purpose: to lengthen and reduce tension in the soleus and assist postural correction.

Preparation

As for the calf stretch, but with feet closer together, body weight central.

Figure 8.53 Standing pectoral stretch

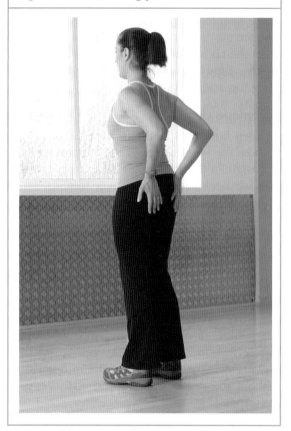

down and lengthen the spine. Feel a stretch across the chest and the front of the shoulders. Repeat as required. Maintain natural breathing.

Technique tips

- Keep the knees soft.
- Open the chest but do not lift it.
- Draw the ribcage down to prevent the back arching.
- Lengthen the spine and keep the neck in line.
- Slide the shoulder blades down.

Standing pectoral stretch

Purpose: to lengthen and reduce tension in the pectoral muscles to assist with postural correction.

Preparation

Stand in correct upright posture, with hands resting on buttocks.

Action

Gently draw in the abdomen and draw the elbows back to open the chest. Draw the ribcage

Figure 8.54 Standing side stretch

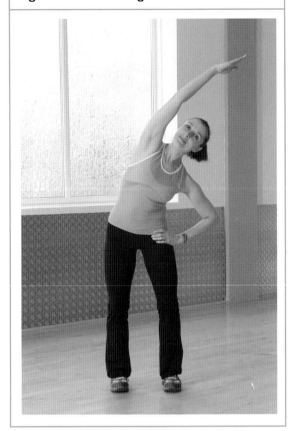

Action

Gently draw in the abdomen and, with the right arm, reach up to the ceiling, lengthening the spine. Continue the lengthening feeling and reach up and over to the left side, sliding the supporting hand down to mid-thigh. Feel a stretch down the right side of body. Lengthen the spine and lift the arm upwards to return to upright position. Lower the arm before repeating on the other side. Maintain natural breathing.

Technique tips

- Continue the upward reach as the body bends to the side.
- Avoid sinking in the supporting side – keep lengthening away.
- Keep the body weight central – avoid pushing the hips out to the side.
- Position the top arm slightly forwards to avoid arching the back.
- Draw the shoulder blades down and lengthen the neck.

Standing side stretch

Purpose: to lengthen and reduce tension in the latissimus dorsi muscles and increase thoracic mobility.

Preparation

Stand in correct upright posture, hands on hips.

Figure 8.55 Standing triceps stretch

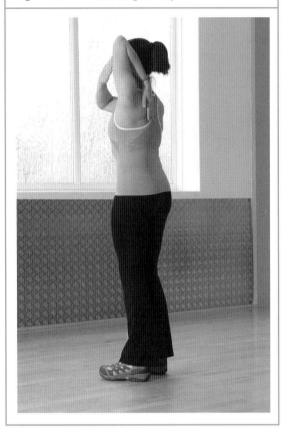

Action

Gently draw in the abdomen and lift the left arm up to the ceiling, bending the elbow and reaching fingers down between the shoulder blades. With the right hand, lengthen the triceps by lifting the elbow towards the ceiling before taking it gently behind the head. Feel the stretch in the back of the left upper arm. Repeat with the other arm. Maintain natural breathing.

Technique tips

- Maintain neutral spine throughout.
- Hinge slightly forwards from the hips to prevent back arching.
- Lift the elbow away from the shoulder.
- Draw the ribcage down to maintain correct spinal alignment.
- If the back begins to arch, try supporting the stretch from the front rather than overhead.
- Keep the head lifted and in line with the spine.
- Slide the shoulder blades down.

Adaptation

This stretch can also be done seated but, for the maintenance of good posture, it is preferable to do it standing.

Standing triceps stretch

Purpose: to lengthen and reduce tension in the triceps to assist postural correction.

Preparation

Stand in correct upright posture.

EXERCISES USING AN UNSTABLE BASE

Working on an unstable base doesn't necessarily make you more stable, but it provides excellent neuromuscular feedback and is useful to educate correct muscle recruitment. Exercises for two types of such equipment – the foam roller and the stability ball – will be discussed next.

> ## Important!
>
> It is important that lumbopelvic stability has been gained before commencing with unstable base equipment and for this reason only *basic* stabilising exercises have been included in this programme. For continuity, these exercises have been categorised into two levels in the same way as described in chapter 3.

This section comprises mostly lumbopelvic stability exercises for the foam roller, but a few additional exercises have been included which are very useful for mobilising stiff areas and for stretching muscles compromised by postural changes.

THE FOAM ROLLER

Introduction to the foam roller

The roller is a fun and versatile tool. It can be used to lie on, supine or prone, to sit on or to place on top of the body. Lying supine on the roller massages the spine, increases circulation and stimulates the discs to absorb fluid. All positions encourage neutral spinal alignment. Pregnancy postural changes can be addressed as the roller helps to identify areas of tightness, weakness and restriction. Prone positions may need adapting for breast comfort.

The following exercises are intended to explore the basic concepts of the roller and introduce the idea to instructors. It is a complex tool to teach but has enormous potential – further training is recommended.

> ## Important!
>
> Once the Level 1 exercises from chapter 3 can be correctly performed on the floor many can be transposed to the roller. Level 2 exercises should not be introduced until Level 1 has been correctly accomplished – progressing too quickly to this level may encourage mis-recruitment of the mobilising muscles.

Supine exercises

Getting into position

The transition from standing to supine lying is an exercise in itself! Since it requires a degree of mobility, flexibility and muscular strength, this position may be inappropriate for some women. *It is particularly unsuitable for women experiencing knee pain and persistent diastasis recti.*

Preparation

Stand in correct upright posture, astride the end of the roller, and clip the ankles either side to keep it in place. Bend the knees and squat down, placing hands on the floor in front to support you. Sit down towards the end of the roller and position it in the crease of the buttocks – this may feel unusual but only requires a brief stay! Move the hands behind you on the floor.

Action

Gently draw in the abdomen, tilt the pelvis and slowly roll down through the spine until you are lying along the roller. Use the arms to assist and do not let the abdomen dome. The aim is to feel each of the vertebrae pressing into the roller during this transition and it may be necessary to tighten the gluteals at the beginning of the movement to get sufficient pelvic tilt to feel the lumbar spine curling down.

Figure 8.56 Getting into position

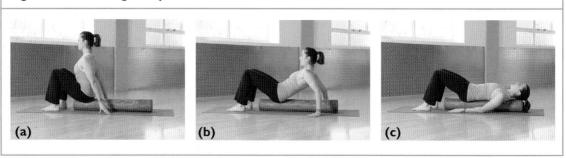

(a)   (b)   (c)

Once in supine position try to get the spine as straight as possible on the surface of the roller and make a mental note of areas that appear to deviate. Rest arms on the floor with palms upwards if possible and relax into the roller, breathing naturally. As the muscles begin to let go, find neutral alignment and allow the body to release further.

NB: This might feel quite uncomfortable initially so it is important to allow a few minutes for your body to settle.

Technique tips

- It is likely that your back will tighten to resist the pressure created by the dense surface of the roller, so it may take some time for the muscles to relax.
- Ensure equal weight on both feet so as not to lean to one side.
- Keep pelvis level.
- Keep chest wide and back of ribcage in contact with the roller.
- Align the head and look up to the ceiling.
- If discomfort is still felt after a few minutes, particularly in the thoracic spine, it may be necessary to put a thin cushion or towel on top of the roller.
- Sacral/coccyx discomfort may be helped by placing a thin sponge or towel underneath the area to reduce pressure.

Caution: Great care should be taken to avoid doming of the abdominals during this transition.

Figure 8.57 Melt down

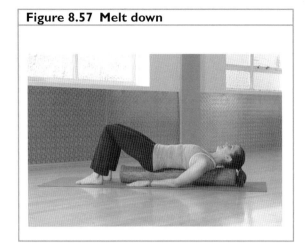

Getting off the foam roller

Moving off the roller may feel a little uncomfortable, particularly if some time has been spent on it. Gently draw in the abdomen and roll the whole body over to the side, as one unit, and push the roller out of the way. Lie back on the floor and enjoy the 'softness' of the new surface. Experience the openness created in the chest and the increased length of the spine. Stay here for a few minutes and relax.

Melt down

Remain in the supine position described above for up to five minutes – the longer the better in order to release unwanted tension. Feel your body slowly giving in to the pressure of the roller and allow the muscles to release. The vertebrae should begin to open and the chest widen as the body melts and becomes one with the support. This is extremely valuable in itself – if there is only time to do this, it will be time well spent.

If time permits, continue to the exercises described below; if not, use the correct procedure to get off the roller.

Figure 8.58 Shoulder release

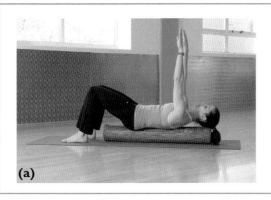

(a)

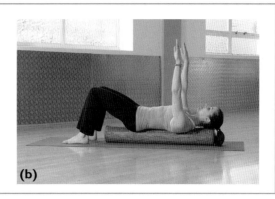

(b)

Shoulder release

Purpose: to release muscular tension and increase thoracic mobility.

Preparation

Lying supine on the roller as above, in correct spinal alignment, float the arms up to the ceiling, one at a time, and relax the shoulder blades down the sides of the roller. Feel as if the arms are suspended from the ceiling.

Action

Recruit TrA first then, as you breathe in, reach up with both arms towards the ceiling, keeping the elbows straight. Feel the shoulder blades lifting around the side of the body and the back of the ribcage sinking further into the roller. Keeping the elbows straight, release the arms and let the shoulder blades melt either side of the roller. Maintain natural breathing.

Technique tips

- Keep arms shoulder-width apart.
- Inhale to lift the arms – this is useful for mobilising the thoracic spine.
- Keep the neck long as the arms lift.
- Let go in the shoulders on the release and allow them to sink further down.
- Feel the shoulder blades relaxing around the roller as you lower.
- Maintain neutral alignment throughout.

Figure 8.59 Chest flye

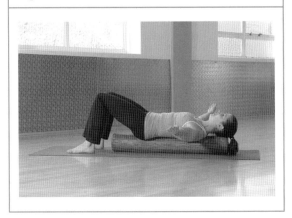

As before, gently drawing in the abdomen to recruit TrA should be cued at the beginning of each exercise and normal breathing encouraged throughout. It is not necessary to give constant reminders to activate TrA – once it has been recruited it should continue to work for the duration of the exercise.

Chest flye

See page 34 for details of this exercise on the floor. It is particularly beneficial to do it on the roller as it helps to lengthen tight pectoral muscles. Pause with the arms open to the sides to allow the muscles to relax and lengthen. This position may induce a nerve stretch, with tingling in the shoulder, down the inside of the arm into the fingers. If this becomes uncomfortable, avoid pausing in position and keep the movement continuous but slow. If postural changes have medially rotated the humerus, the range of movement may be reduced and nerve impingement may occur. Encouraging lateral rotation of the humerus prior to the exercise will be beneficial.

The following additional Level 1 exercises from chapter 3 can be switched to the roller, *provided they can be correctly performed on the floor.*

- Scissor arms
- Arm circle
- Pelvic tilt
- Leg slide
- Leg slide with scissor arms/arm circle/chest flye
- Knee raise
- Spine curl – range of movement is reduced on the roller

Tabletop at the wall

This position requires increased use of the global stabilisers to stay on the roller! *It is inappropriate for women recovering from PGP due to the awkward transition.*

Moving into tabletop at the wall

Depending on the length of the roller, one end can be positioned against the wall. Shorter rollers should be further away. Move carefully into position as follows – this is more difficult due to reduced space for the knees! Lie supine on the roller as before in correct spinal alignment, with arms resting on the floor for added support. Recruit TrA and float one leg up to rest on the wall; repeat with the other leg. Position the feet hip-width apart, with a 90-degree angle at the knees and hips. If this position is uncomfortable for the lower back, move into imprinted tabletop as discussed on page 40. Release the hip flexors and allow the legs to rest gently on the wall. Draw the ribcage gently down and lengthen the spine.

Use the following two exercises as an introduction to the position, using the wall for support.

Figure 8.62 Scapular stabilisation

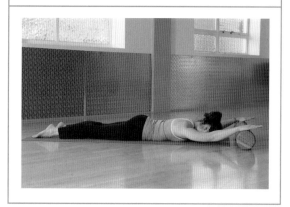

Prone exercises

This position may not be comfortable for breast-feeding mums. Pressure may be relieved by placing rolled up towels or soft cushions above and below the breasts; if discomfort persists, these exercises may have to be postponed.

Scapular stabilisation

Purpose: to strengthen the lower trapezius to provide shoulder stabilisation and improve upper body posture.

Preparation

Lie prone with legs together and arms reaching above the head in a wide V, close to the ends of the roller. Position the roller firmly under-neath the heel of the hand and draw the shoulder blades down your back. Lift the elbows off the floor and relax the forehead to the floor or on a small cushion.

Action

Recruit TrA first then inhale and slowly roll the roller downwards so it moves from the heel of the hand to the fingertips. Keep the elbows almost straight so that the movement comes from the shoulder blades, which should slide further down the back. On the return phase, draw the shoulder blades down to resist the upward pull and keep the neck long. Maintain natural breathing.

Technique tips

- Keep the movement small but well controlled.
- Focus on drawing the shoulder blades down during both phases of the movement.
- Keep the wrists lifted.
- Keep the torso still – draw ribs to hips to maintain alignment.
- If the back feels uncomfortable, place a small cushion underneath the abdomen.

Figure 8.63 Scapular stabilisation with thoracic extension

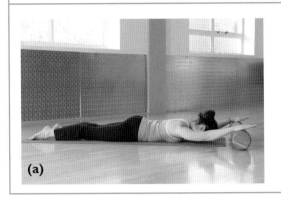

(a)

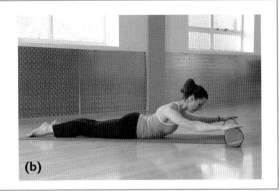

(b)

Scapular stabilisation with thoracic extension

Draw the roller downwards as for scapular stabilisation above and continue the movement by lifting the upper body to extend the thoracic spine. Maintain connection between ribs and hips and keep the movement only in the thoracic spine. Do not allow the lower back to hyperextend. This is an excellent exercise to correct kyphotic posture.

Figure 8.64 Kneeling leg and arm raise

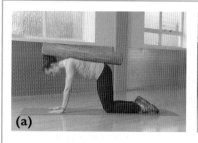 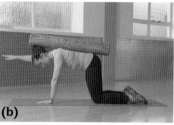 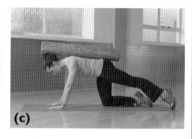

(a) (b) (c)

Kneeling leg and arm raise

With the roller balanced along the spine in a kneeling position, perform the kneeling leg and arm exercise as described on page 39. Build up to the complete exercise in the following stages:

- Arm lift
- Leg slide
- Arm lift and leg slide together
- Leg lift
- Arm lift and leg lift together

Correct spinal alignment in kneeling

The roller is a very useful tool to check correct alignment in kneeling. Place the roller lengthways along the spine and try to balance it there. Points of contact should be sacrum, lower ribs and back of head. Good alignment will enable the roller to remain there for longer!

Stretching on the roller adds an extra stability factor as it encourages the continued use of the deep stabilising muscles. Seated hamstring and gluteal stretches, as described on pages 131–132, can be performed seated sideways on the roller, taking care not to let the knees hyperextend.

Figure 8.65 Roller pectoral stretch

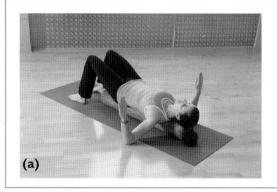
(a)

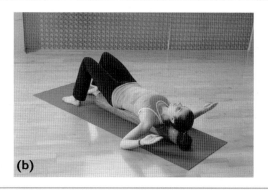
(b)

Stretches

Stretching on the roller adds an extra stability factor as it encourages the continued use of the deep stabilising muscles.

Roller hamstring stretch

Sit sideways on the roller and perform seated hamstring stretch as described on page 131, taking care not to allow the knees to hyperextend.

Roller gluteal stretch

Sit sideways on the roller and perform the seated gluteal stretch as described on page 132, taking care not to allow the knees to hyperextend.

Roller pectoral stretch

Purpose: to lengthen and reduce tension in pectoralis minor for improved posture and increased shoulder mobility.

Preparation

Lie supine on the roller, with feet on the floor and spine in correct alignment. Rest the arms on the floor to the sides at shoulder height and bend the elbows to 90 degrees, with forearms vertical and palms pointing towards the feet.

Action

Inhale to prepare and as you exhale recruit TrA and slowly lower the forearms and back of hand to the floor towards the head, keeping the elbows on the floor and wrist/forearms aligned. Ensure that the ribcage stays into the roller. Hold the position at its furthest point, continuing to breathe, and try to relax.

Technique tips

- Maintain neutral spinal alignment.
- Do not allow the ribcage to lift.
- Allow the arms to relax – avoid hanging on.
- Aim to get the wrist to the floor.

Figure 8.66 Seated posture

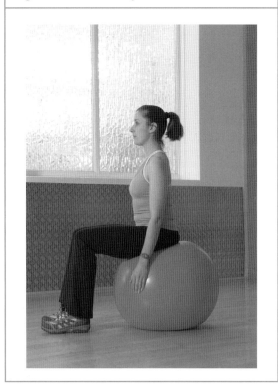

THE STABILITY BALL

This section contains basic lumbopelvic stability exercises along with a few additional exercises for mobility and stretching. It also includes additional exercises for training muscular endurance.

Introduction to the stability ball

Once lumbopelvic stability has been gained, the ball provides an excellent base for training the postural muscles in sitting. The adoption of correct upright seated posture on the ball aids recruitment of TrA and the PFM. Not only does slumped sitting switch off the deep stabilising muscles, it also increases the ball's instability.

> ## Important!
> The following is a small selection of suitable postnatal exercises on the ball, which build in intensity and complexity. As before, Level I exercises should be fully accomplished before progressing to the more challenging Level 2 exercises. Further training on the ball is recommended for the inexperienced instructor.

Level 1: Seated exercises

Seated posture

Purpose: to redress posture in sitting and improve lumbopelvic stability.

Preparation

Ensure that the ball is the correct size for you and inflated sufficiently – incorrect size will cause misalignment of the knees and hips. Place feet hip-width apart, flat on the floor, with a 90-degree angle at the hips and the knees. Rest hands on thighs or on the ball.

Action

Sit for a few minutes, breathing naturally and maintaining correct body alignment. Unsupported sitting is an endurance activity, so don't overdo it!

Technique tips
- Distribute weight equally on both feet.
- Position yourself directly on your sit bones.
- Lengthen the spine away from bones.
- Maintain neutral spinal alignment.
- Slide the shoulder blades down.

NB: You may need to begin with feet a little wider than hip-width to help you balance. Narrowing the width of your base will reduce stability and make the exercises more challenging.

Figure 8.67 Seated pelvic tilt

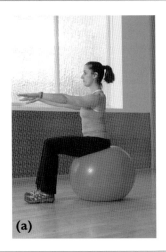
(a)

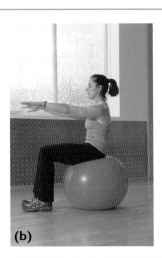
(b)

Seated pelvic tilt

Purpose: to shorten RA and improve lumbopelvic stability.

Preparation

Start seated as above, hands reaching forwards for balance.

Action

Inhale to prepare and as you exhale recruit TrA and tilt the pelvis, lifting the pubic bone up towards the breast bone. Use the abdominals rather than the buttocks to create the movement and allow the ball to roll underneath you. Release and return to upright sitting, rolling the ball back. Maintain natural breathing.

Figure 8.68 Seated hip circle

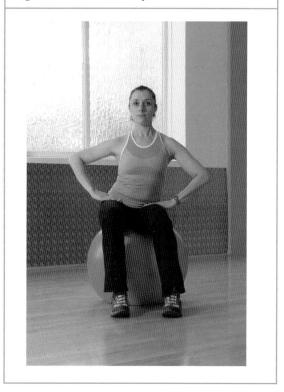

Action

Move through the pelvic tilt and continue the hips around in a circle. Make the movement as large as possible but avoid slumping into an anterior tilt. Return to the upright seated position and lift away from the sit bones. Repeat in the other direction.

Seated hip circle

Purpose: to loosen the lower back.

Preparation

Start seated as above.

Figure 8.69 Seated heel raise

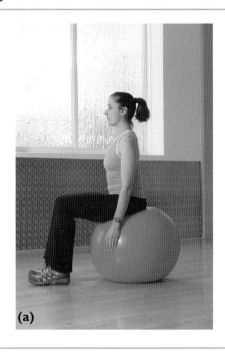

(a)

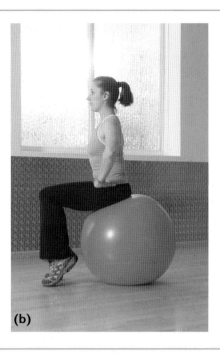

(b)

Seated heel raise

Purpose: to mobilise the feet and improve lumbopelvic stability.

Preparation

Start seated as above.

Action

Inhale to prepare and as you exhale recruit TrA and lift the heels, rolling the ball forwards. Pause before rolling back. Maintain natural breathing.

Technique tips

- Maintain upright sitting throughout.
- Lift the arches of the feet as high as possible with weight travelling through the centre of each foot and equally distributed across the toe joints.

Progression

To develop into a strengthening exercise for the calves, lean the upper body forwards and rest hands or elbows on thighs.

Figure 8.70 Seated knee raise

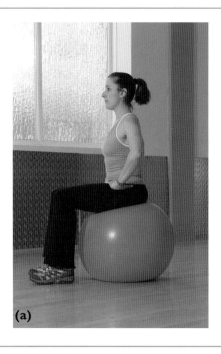

(a)

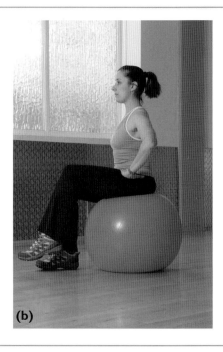

(b)

Seated knee raise

Purpose: to improve lumbopelvic stability.

Preparation

Seated as above.

Action

Inhale to prepare and as you exhale recruit TrA and transfer the weight onto the left foot. Float the right leg off the floor and lift the knee. Pause before lowering and transfer weight onto the right foot. Repeat with alternate legs. Maintain natural breathing.

Technique tips

- Maintain upright sitting and lift away from sit bones.
- Avoid pushing down onto the supporting foot.
- Avoid lifting the hip with the knee.
- Keep the weight centred across both sit bones – do not lean onto the supporting side.
- Perform slowly to encourage the stabilising muscles to work for longer.

Figure 8.71 Seated scissor arms

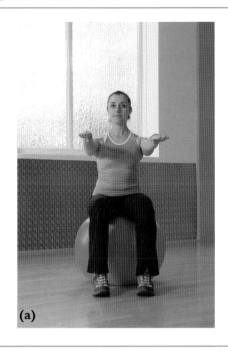

(a)

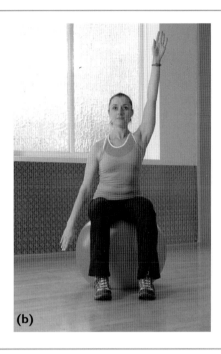

(b)

Seated scissor arms

Purpose: to improve lumbopelvic stability.

Preparation

Seated as above, but with arms lifted up in front at chest height, shoulders relaxed.

Action

Inhale to prepare and as you exhale recruit TrA and lift one arm up above the head and lower the other down by your side, sliding the shoulder of the top arm down. Keeping the arms straight, slowly float both arms back to chest height and repeat, changing arms. Maintain natural breathing.

Technique tips

- Lift away from your sit bones.
- Maintain upright sitting as the arm lifts.
- Draw the ribcage down as the arm lifts
- Lengthen both arms as far away from the shoulders as possible.
- Slide the shoulder blades down your back throughout.
- Keep the movement slow and controlled.

Figure 8.72 Seated scissor arms with knee raise

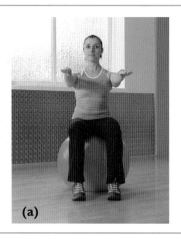

(a)

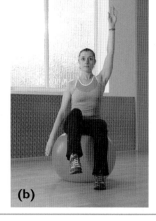

(b)

Seated scissor arms with knee raise

Purpose: to improve lumbopelvic stability – this exercise requires increased assistance from the global stabilisers.

Preparation

Seated as above, with arms lifted up in front at chest height, shoulders relaxed.

Action

Combine the scissor arms and knee raise exercises described above.

Technique tips

- Maintain upright sitting throughout.
- Avoid pressing down into the supporting foot.
- Peel the foot off the floor and float the knee up.
- Keep the ribcage and shoulder blades drawn down.
- Lengthen both arms as far away from the shoulders as possible.
- Keep the transition smooth.
- Avoid lifting the hip with the knee.
- Keep the weight centred across both sit bones – do not lean onto the supporting side.
- Lift away from your sit bones.
- Keep the movement slow and controlled.

Figure 8.73 Prone arm raise

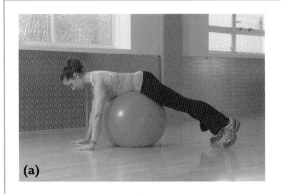

(a)

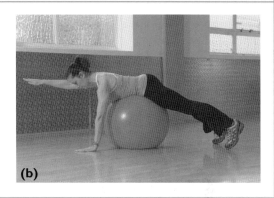

(b)

Level 1: Prone exercises

Prone balance position on the stability ball

This position may not be comfortable for women with heavy breasts or caesarean scars! It may also not be appropriate immediately after eating or with a full bladder! Deflating the ball a little may increase comfort.

Lie over the ball, with hands flat on the floor and toes curled under the feet. Ensure that equal weight is distributed between these four points. The breasts should be just off the ball. Push down through the hands to lift out of the shoulders, keeping the elbows soft. Lengthen the legs out of the hips and soften the knees. Feel the head and tailbone lengthening away in opposite directions and slide the shoulder blades down.

Prone arm raise

Purpose: to strengthen lower trapezius for postural correction and improve lumbopelvic stability.

Preparation

Lie on the ball in the prone balance position.

Action

Inhale to prepare and while exhaling recruit TrA and transfer the upper body weight onto the left side. Float the right arm off the floor and reach forwards above the head at shoulder height. Keep the head aligned – do not allow it to hyperextend. Lower and transfer upper body weight onto the right side. Repeat, alternating sides. Maintain natural breathing.

Technique tips

- Lift away from the ball – do not allow the abdomen to sink down as this will compromise the back.
- Lengthen the arm away from the shoulder.
- Push down through the supporting hand to avoid sinking into the shoulder.
- Draw the shoulder blades down.
- Keep the torso square.
- Keep the other three supports firmly on the floor.
- Maintain neutral alignment throughout.

Progression

Move the body weight further forwards onto the hands.

Figure 8.74 Gluteal raise

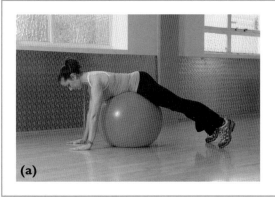

(a)

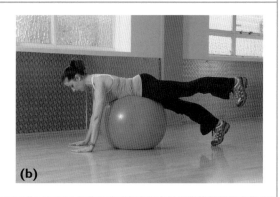

(b)

Gluteal raise

Purpose: to strengthen gluteus maximus for postural correction and improve lumbopelvic stability.

Preparation

Assume the prone balance position.

Action

Inhale to prepare and as you exhale recruit TrA and transfer the lower body weight onto the left side. Tighten the gluteals and float the right leg off the floor, lengthening the leg away from the hip. Do not allow the back to hyperextend. Lower and transfer the lower body weight onto the right side. Repeat, alternating sides. Maintain natural breathing.

Technique tips

- Tighten the gluteals prior to lifting to encourage correct muscle recruitment.
- Lift away from the ball – do not allow the abdomen to sink down as this will compromise the back.
- Push down through the hands to avoid sinking into the shoulder.
- Draw the shoulder blades down.
- Keep the torso square and hips on the ball.
- Keep the other three supports firmly on the floor.
- Maintain neutral alignment throughout.
- Alternating legs increases the stabilisation challenge.

Figure 8.75 Swimming

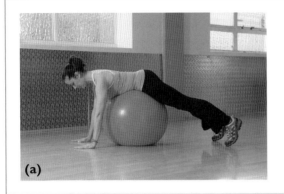

(a)

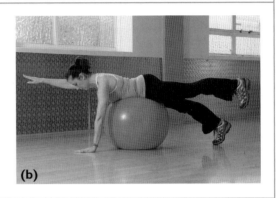

(b)

Swimming

Purpose: to strengthen gluteus maximus and lower trapezius for postural correction and improve lumbopelvic stability.

This is a combination of the two previous exercises, i.e. an arm raise and an opposite gluteal raise.

Preparation

Assume the prone balance position, but with hands and feet opened wider to the side for added stability.

Action

Inhale to prepare and as you exhale recruit TrA and slowly lift right arm and left leg as in the two exercises described above. Pause and lengthen the limbs away from the centre. Lower and repeat, alternating sides. Maintain natural breathing.

Technique tips

As for the above exercises, plus:
- Feel a diagonal reach from fingers through to opposite toes.
- Keep the head aligned with spine.
- Lift through the ribcage to maintain correct alignment.
- Keep the transition smooth and controlled.

Progression

Narrow the base by bringing feet in to hip-width apart and hands to shoulder-width apart. This reduces stability and makes the exercise more challenging.

Figure 8.78 Press-up

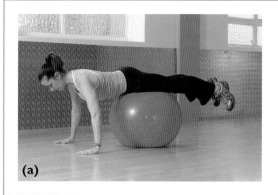

(a)

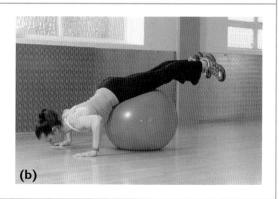

(b)

Press-up

Purpose: to strengthen pectorals and triceps for lifting and carrying and to increase lumbopelvic stability.

Preparation

From prone balance position with legs together, walk the hands forwards so the legs are lifted parallel to the floor and the ball is centred under the hips. Keep arms straight, with hands wider than shoulders and fingers facing forwards. Draw the shoulder blades down and lengthen the spine.

Action

Inhale to prepare and as you exhale recruit TrA and bend the elbows to lower the upper body towards the floor, keeping the head aligned with the spine. Keeping the body weight forwards, slowly straighten the elbows and return to the starting position. Maintain natural breathing.

Technique tips

- Maintain neutral alignment throughout.
- Push down through the hands to avoid sinking into the shoulders.
- Slide the shoulder blades down your back.
- Check elbows remain over wrists while bending.
- Avoid flexing the elbows below 90 degrees.
- Don't lock out the elbows as they extend.
- Keep the head aligned with the spine.

Caution: If the stabilising muscles are weak, the spine will sag and the back may be compromised. In such cases this exercise should be postponed until appropriate strength has been gained.

Progression

Walk the hands further forwards so the ball rolls onto the thighs. Lengthening the lever in this way increases the workload on the prime movers and stabilising muscles.

Figure 8.79 Stability ball squat

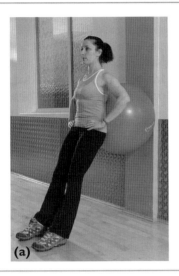

(a)

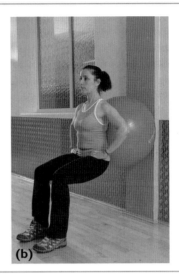

(b)

Level 2: Standing exercise

Stability ball squat

Purpose: to strengthen gluteus maximus, hamstrings and quadriceps for postural correction and increase lumbopelvic stability.

Preparation

Stand in correct upright posture at the wall, with the ball positioned between the lower back and the wall. Walk the feet out one or two paces and position them hip-width apart. Place hands on hips or relaxed by sides and lean back onto the ball keeping the spine aligned.

Action

Inhale to prepare and while exhaling recruit TrA and slowly squat down, keeping the spine lifted as the ball rolls up your back. Tighten the gluteals and drive slowly back to upright posture, straightening the knees. Maintain natural breathing.

Technique tips

- Maintain upright posture throughout.
- Avoid flexing the knees below 90 degrees.
- Drop the tailbone straight down towards the floor.
- Keep knees tracking over toes as you bend.
- Press down through the heels to straighten up.
- Avoid locking out the knees as they extend.
- Keep the upper body lifted.
- Lean into the ball.

Progression

Increase the length of hold at the lowest point of the squat, maintaining alignment as above.

routine of an organised new mum. If undertaken on a regular basis the duration need only be 10 minutes. Less frequent sessions would require a longer duration in order to gain similar benefits. A previously fit woman, on the other hand, may attempt to return immediately to her pre-pregnancy training regime in a desperate attempt to regain her previous shape. This should be discouraged as the effects of pregnancy and delivery will have taken a greater toll on her body than may be realised, and there is a strong possibility that overexertion in the early weeks will impede recovery. CV training should build up to the optimum three sessions per week but should not exceed five. The risks involved with more frequent exercise may outweigh the potential benefits. Rest is essential for a new mum and a period of relaxation should be structured into the day in exactly the same way that exercise is.

What intensity is recommended?

Similar aerobic benefits can be achieved by performing high-intensity/short-duration exercise as can be achieved by low-intensity/long-duration exercise, but the latter is a much more suitable option. Gentle to moderate intensity is recommended in the early weeks, progressing to a moderate level as energy increases. An RPE of 4–6 is recommended (see Appendix). The 'talk test' provides a realistic guide to the level of work.

How long should the session last?

Commencing with 10 minutes of cardiovascular work (not including warm-up and cool-down) should be sufficient to gain small benefits if performed a few times a week. Less frequent sessions would require a longer duration. This could gradually increase to 20 and up to 30 minutes, provided the intensity is kept to a moderate level. Incorporating periods of active rest into the workout will prevent it becoming too demanding. A further factor for consideration is local muscular endurance, which will shorten the duration if fatigue sets in. Continuing over an extended period of time also increases the risk of injury to the joints and pelvic floor.

Types of cardiovascular training

A variety of CV activities are available, some more suitable than others, for postnatal women. The optimum three sessions a week should ideally comprise different activities, e.g. a brisk walk with baby, a swim and a session on the bike. Activities should be introduced individually on separate occasions so that, should problems develop, the cause can be more easily identified. Studio-based cardiovascular activities are discussed in chapter 11.

Gait

This relates to the pattern of movement of the limbs and is a continuum from slow walking to fast running. It involves the three major joints of the lower body – ankle, knee and hip – working together with the pelvis, spine and upper limbs. The effects of pregnancy on joint stability, alignment, reduced lumbopelvic stability and biomechanical changes have significant implications for gait. The factors in table 9.1 should be considered before a walking or jogging programme is undertaken.

Table 9.1	Factors to consider before undertaking a walking or jogging programme
	Factors
Foot	Dropped arches, toeing out and ankle eversion (rolling in) reduce ankle stability, change the action of the foot and compromise absorption of ground forces. Poor foot alignment also reduces the propulsive forces from the big toe that are necessary for effective calf muscle functioning. This is particularly relevant postnatally, as the calves help to reduce oedema and improve blood flow through varicose veins. Weak dorsiflexors may contribute to the poor rolling action of the foot. The dissipation of ground force through the foot is crucial for the safety of the joints above, so correct foot placement is vital. An everted ankle joint will reduce pelvic stability as it unlocks the SIJ.
Leg	The forward shift in centre of gravity increases the activity of the calves, making them more vulnerable to cramping. Increased tension in the calves, together with weakened tibialis anterior, reduces the dorsiflexion action of the ankle.
Thigh	Weight gain, reduced ligamentous support and changes in the Q angle affect the stability of the knee. Muscle imbalance between vastus medialis/lateralis, due to the change in the angle of the thigh, reduces the output of the quadriceps group and may compromise the biomechanics of the knee joint. The possible displacement of the head of the femur into the front of the acetabulum, caused by the pull of tight deep lateral rotators, affects joint action and alignment.
Pelvis	Muscle imbalance between shortened iliopsoas and poor muscle tone in gluteus maximus reduce stride length and potential for forward drive. Reduced pelvic stability from weakened gluteus medius and external obliques increases lateral sway and vulnerability of SP and SIJ. Tight erector spinae and reduced thoracic mobility result in whole trunk rotation on weight transference and lack of spinal flow. See chapter 2 for further discussion on reduced lumbopelvic stability.

Guidelines for a cardiovascular session

- Spend time mobilising all joints to ensure effective loosening.
- Consider postural adaptation and individual comfort when selecting suitable equipment.
- Pulse raise on a different piece of equipment to the main workout to vary joint and muscle action.
- Use dynamic rather than static stretching.
- Vary the use of equipment wherever possible.
- Maintain correct spinal alignment and exercise technique throughout.

- Ensure warm-down provides sufficient time for breathing and heart rate recovery.
- Allow sufficient time to stretch all muscles worked as well as those affected by postural changes.
- Stretch to *maintain muscle length* not to increase flexibility.

CARDIOVASCULAR ACTIVITIES

Buggy pushing

This is an excellent activity as it can easily be incorporated into a new lifestyle with baby. A brisk walk around the park needs no special equipment, apart from a suitable sturdy buggy, and can be undertaken at any convenient time. However, in addition to posture and gait, consideration should be given to the suitability of the buggy, as an unsuitable model may compromise postural recovery. There are numerous buggies on the market offering a variety of designs but if new mums are intending to incorporate buggy pushing into their fitness regime, the following points should be considered for a buggy's suitability:

- **Stability:** While a lightweight buggy can be very versatile it becomes quite unstable when pushed 'off-road'. If the local stabilising muscles are weak, additional support is needed from the global stabilisers, which may already be over-recruiting. The absence of storage underneath the seat may necessitate bags being carried over the buggy handles; not only will this affect stability but it also compromises posture (*see* key points below).
- **Handle height**: A handle which is too low may induce additional kyphosis if it requires women to stoop forwards, while a handle that is too high will elevate the shoulders and may distort wrist alignment.
- **Handle type:** A horizontal handlebar, held with an overhand grip, medially rotates the humerus and encourages a more kyphotic posture, whereas handles on a cantilever buggy place the humerus in a more appropriate position.
- **Rear wheel framework:** A horizontal bar positioned between the two back wheels will dictate stride length if the mum's feet catch on the bar. In order to lengthen the stride, mums will naturally walk to the side of the buggy, holding with one hand only, or they will hinge forwards from the hips and push with their upper body leaning forwards. Both of these adaptations are unsuitable: pushing the buggy with one hand stresses the wrist and elbow and increases the likelihood of tendonitis, and taking the hips back compromises correct posture and reduces the support from the local stabilising muscles. This stance is also adopted if bags are carried on the handles.

Key points
- Maintain correct postural alignment and walk tall.
- Use a heel-toe action to roll through the foot.
- Push off from the big toe and lift the arch of the foot.
- Drive back with the heel to push forwards and work into the gluteals.
- Keep knees aligned – avoid rolling in.
- Keep the hips level and avoid dipping from side to side.
- Relax the elbows and let them drop into the sides of the body.
- Draw the shoulder blades down and open the chest.
- Hold the buggy handle with a relaxed grip – preferably at the side of the frame.

Uphill pushing frequently demonstrates the need to strengthen gluteus maximus – as seen in the forwards leaning, head down, straight arm push! This slumped posture switches off the local stabilising muscles and increases the downward pressure onto the pelvic floor. Walking tall, keeping hips close to handles and driving forwards with the buttocks should be encouraged. Rolling the hips side to side during uphill or downhill pushing should also be discouraged and strengthening exercises for gluteus medius commenced.

Buggy-free walking

Walking without baby offers a potentially more effective workout as the upper body can be employed in the activity and correct postural alignment maintained. Spinal alignment should be corrected if heavy breasts pull the upper body forwards, although an over-compensated, leaning back position will increase stress on the lumbar spine. Excessive pelvic movement may occur when the pace increases as the body weight rocks from side to side; this should be avoided if pelvic girdle problems persist.

Outdoor walking offers the benefits of fresh air, adequate cooling for the body, and sunlight, which provides vitamin D – essential for the absorption of calcium (*see* page 69). Variable terrain walking provides intensity changes, but may increase the risk of incorrect joint alignment. Adherence to correct technique is vital, particularly when speed increases and pelvic movement becomes more accentuated. The following key points, additional to those for buggy pushing, apply to treadmill or outdoor walking.

Key points (additional to those above)

- Take long, comfortable strides.
- Relax the shoulders and open the chest.
- Let the arms swing naturally from the shoulders.

Caution: If PGP is experienced, this activity should be stopped and an alternative method of training adopted.

Nordic walking

Under the guidance of a qualified Nordic walking instructor this is an excellent low-impact, whole-body activity for postnatal women. Correct use of the poles encourages upright posture and enhances a rolling foot action during gait. As stride length increases, the front of the hips open and activation of gluteus maximus is enhanced. Increased support provided by the poles puts a spring in the step and allows the body to lift from the hips; this reduces lateral sway during the stance phase and encourages activation of gluteus medius.

The action of the arms will help to lengthen tight pectorals and strengthen latissimus dorsi during the backward drive. Assuming lumbopelvic stability has been achieved, the added bonus of the arm action is that it encourages a degree of trunk rotation, and this will increase thoracic mobility and activate the obliques to stabilise the torso. Breasts need to be well supported to reduce movement, and feeding before exercise is essential. Correct technique should help to release tension in the neck and shoulders but close observation is necessary to prevent aggravating the situation. Relaxed shoulders and an upright head position should be encouraged throughout. Walking on uneven terrain improves balance, stability and bone density.

Jogging

Jogging increases the stress to the joints, breasts and PFM. An elevated running style (bounce) and poor foot action, often adopted by inexperienced runners, further increases the load, which, together with reduced lumbopelvic stability, is the reason why newcomers should be discouraged from running too soon. Experienced runners, demonstrating good technique and minimum vertical action, should only recommence when they have regained lumbopelvic stability. This timeframe is very individual!

To reduce the impact when running outdoors choose softer surfaces rather than concrete paths or tarmac, and keep a shorter stride length to avoid a heavy heel strike. Variable terrain does, however, require greater input from the global stabilisers to maintain balance and increases the vulnerability of the knees and ankles.

Running on a treadmill with split-level belts may encourage increased lateral sway if gluteus medius is unable to provide sufficient support.

Key points

- Wear a bra that provides sufficient support for the breasts and reduces the bounce.
- Select appropriate footwear, preferably a running shoe designed to absorb the shock through the heel and support the ankle joint.
- Maintain good postural alignment.
- Adapt the stride length for comfort.
- Aim for a heel strike directly under the knee.
- Use a heel-toe action to roll through the foot.
- Push off from the big toe and lift the arch of the foot.
- Keep knees aligned – avoid rolling in.
- Relax the shoulders and open the chest.
- Bend the elbows and keep them close to the body.
- Allow a gentle forwards and backwards arm motion.

Uphill running

- Shorten the stride and encourage forefoot strike.
- Lean slightly forwards from the hip.

Downhill running

- Keep the feet under the body.
- Lean gently forwards into the hill – avoid leaning backwards.
- Keep lateral pelvic movement to a minimum.

Jogging with the buggy

This is an inappropriate activity and has implications for the safety of both mother and baby – even with a buggy specifically designed for this purpose. In addition to the effects of biomechanical changes on gait, the presence of the buggy further compromises posture and gait. The four key points discussed in buggy walking are magnified, as speed and stride length increase and one-handed pushing is adopted to enable a longer stride. This has implications for wrist, forearm, shoulder and spinal alignment, with the resulting rotated gait, particularly in the thoracic spine, exacerbating muscle imbalances.

Lack of adequate suspension means that baby may be subjected to all the bumps and vibrations of the terrain, and the risks increase further if running off-road with obstacles such as tree roots and fallen branches to contend with! Due to the lack of head support provided in jogging buggies, most manufacturers recommend that these are only suitable for use with babies aged at least six months – many women will ignore such warnings.

Instructors conducting this type of session should consider their professional responsibility under their legal duty of care to both mother and baby. Even though the mother is present in the session, the instructor may also be liable in relation to the long-term well-being of the baby as a result of activities, which were recommended or condoned by a fitness professional, where the baby was present. Most insurance companies will not cover instructors to teach this activity. (*See* chapter 14 for further discussion on this.)

Breathing

Newcomers to running frequently experience problems with their breathing, i.e. holding their breath or becoming preoccupied with it, and being unsure when to breathe. This will obviously affect their performance. The diaphragm has two functions: not only is it a muscle of respiration but it is also one of the deep four stabilisers responsible for supporting the spine. During running, the force of the foot strike destabilises the body, and the muscles of the inner unit must respond to maintain balance and support. Untrained muscles will be unable to cope with respiration and stabilisation for long and will fatigue much quicker. Lumbopelvic stability is reduced after respiratory fatigue and this increases the risk of injury.

Cadence breathing

This technique is recommended as it's easy to use but may need a little practice as it involves breathing that is synchronised with the dominant foot strike, e.g. breathe in when the right foot strikes the ground and breathe out when it strikes again. As mums become more competent they could develop this further by using different points of the running stride, such as heel strike or toe off, to adapt their own breathing pattern.

Cycling

Although body weight is supported during cycling and there is no impact to the breasts and PFM, there are still factors to be considered. The saddle of an upright bike may lack support for widened sit bones, and the nose of the seat may be quite painful for a sore perineum or for the SP. The forwards leaning position also exacerbates kyphotic changes in the thoracic spine.

The recumbent bike offers a more comfortable ride but, as the name suggests, does encourage slumping and this will affect activation of TrA and the PFM. Placing a cushion in the back of the seat may improve spinal alignment but this may affect joint angle and action, and reduce comfort. Limited duration is recommended for these reasons. Seat positioning is crucial to avoid stress to the pelvis and knees: one that is too far forward may place excessive strain on the knees and one that is too far back requires the pelvis to shift from side to side in order to extend the knee effectively. A comfortable seated position should allow the knees to extend but not lock out and the pelvis should remain still. The elevated leg position of the recumbent bike is particularly beneficial for improved circulation and venous return but it does rely heavily on the endurance of the quadriceps and hamstrings, and local muscle fatigue may limit duration. Studio cycling is discussed in chapter 11.

Key points

- Maintain correct neutral alignment and sit tall.
- Keep knees aligned – avoid rolling in.
- Keep pelvis still throughout.
- Relax the shoulders and open the chest.
- If the hips are shifting side to side, the seat is incorrectly positioned.

Caution: Stop immediately if pain is felt in the pelvis or knee joint.

Rowing machine

Stationary rowing is a highly co-ordinated and disciplined activity. Working both the upper and lower body, rowing requires high levels of motor skills to perform safely and effectively. It is only suitable for postnatal women who had experience of this equipment before their pregnancy and have regained lumbopelvic stability – even then, the rowing sequence may need to be retrained. The risk of leaning too far back makes this activity unsuitable for inexperienced rowers and large breasts will reduce the range of movement. Weak, inactive stabilising muscles will be unable to maintain adequate support for the spine, necessitating the recruitment of RA, and doming may occur. Rowing should not be reintroduced to the experienced rower too soon.

NB: It is unlikely that this equipment will have been used during pregnancy due to the severely decreased range of movement caused by the bump!

Key points

- Maintain correct neutral alignment and sit tall.
- Keep knees aligned – avoid rolling in.
- Draw the shoulder blades down and keep the chest open.
- Avoid locking elbows or knees.
- Keep the arms close to the body.
- Keep the back in an upright position – do not lean back.
- Do not slump forwards during the return phase.

Caution: Leaning back with poor lumbopelvic stability may cause doming or back pain; do not allow the knees to hyperextend.

Stepping machines

Stepping is a fully weight-bearing activity of moderate impact, demanding a high degree of pelvic movement. An effective workout requires full range of movement, but this may place too much stress on the SIJ and SP as the pelvis rocks from side to side with each downward movement. Range of movement can be reduced by taking shallow steps, which will reduce lateral sway, but this may be hard to sustain over a prolonged period of time and may still irritate lax SIJ. Heavy breasts may pull the body forwards so it may be necessary to hold on to the handrails to maintain correct upright posture. This supported position will reduce the effectiveness of the workout but may provide a welcome break. Pace should be moderate; speeding up may not give the knees sufficient time to extend or cause them to lock out. Local muscle fatigue will determine the duration of this activity.

Key points

- Maintain correct neutral alignment and stand tall.
- Avoid locking out the knees.
- Keep knees aligned – avoid rolling in.
- Relax the shoulders and open the chest.

- Keep the back lifted with a slight forward lean – hold the handrails for support if required.
- Keep the head in line and avoid looking down at the feet.

Caution: Do not allow the knee joints to lock out; avoid excessive pelvic movement.

Cross-trainers

Many of the concerns of stepping machines are reduced with the elliptical leg action of a cross-trainer as this is less stressful to the pelvis. A cross-training machine with handles requires the co-ordinated use of the upper and lower body, which has greater cardiovascular benefits than a machine without. It does, however, require good lumbopelvic stability to prevent excessive pelvic rotation. For this reason it is recommended to postpone the involvement of the upper body until appropriate stability has been gained. Unsupported walking has the additional benefit of improving balance. Footplates that include a lateral motion are inappropriate for postnatal women.

Key points (additional to those for the stepper)

- Hold the bars at elbow height with loose grip.
- Encourage a smooth, natural stride length.
- Allow the torso to roll in a fluid motion.
- Keep the elbows as close to the body as possible.
- Draw the shoulder blades down and allow a gentle forward and backward arm motion.
- Add intervals of increased upper body work.

Swimming

This is an excellent activity and can be commenced when bleeding and discharge has completely finished. The buoyancy of the water eliminates stress to the joints and pelvic floor and reduces the weight of the breasts. It also has additional relaxing qualities and, provided the water temperature is not too cold, can be very therapeutic. Breaststroke is the most leisurely stroke, although the spine may be at risk of hyperextension if the head is held too high out of the water. This stroke may also be unsuitable if pelvic girdle pain has been experienced, as the wide abduction and adduction of the legs may aggravate the condition. Front crawl and backstroke, however, require vigorous arm movements, which may encourage milk flow. The demanding, highly physical action of butterfly should be confined to the very fit, experienced swimmer. Further discussion can be found in chapter 12.

SUMMARY

- Regular CV exercise of the appropriate frequency, intensity, duration and type is beneficial to postnatal recovery and may assist weight loss.
- Low-impact activities are recommended and correct joint alignment is essential.
- High-impact activities will stress the joints, pelvic floor and breasts.
- Decreased joint stability increases the likelihood of injury.
- Improvement in lumbopelvic stability is essential to maintain control in CV activities.
- Co-ordinated arm and leg movements require stronger abdominal stabilisation.
- The breasts should be well supported with an appropriate sports bra or two.
- Vigorous arm movements may cause the breasts to leak.
- Feed or express before commencing activity.
- Moderate-intensity training and good hydration will not affect milk quality or quantity.
- Training should build up to three sessions a week but should not exceed five.
- Intensity should be gentle to moderate during

the early weeks, progressing to a moderate level as energy increases.
- An RPE of 4–6 is recommended.
- Duration can be gradually increased from 10 minutes to 20–30 minutes, depending on the intensity of the workout.
- Brisk walks with baby can be integrated into the daily routine.
- Outdoor walking is particularly beneficial for assisting calcium absorption.
- Activities requiring repetitive joint action may increase discomfort.
- Gait changes should be assessed before a walking or jogging programme is undertaken.
- Correct running style is essential to reduce risks.
- Running with the buggy is unsafe and inappropriate.
- A slumped sitting posture switches off the local stabilising muscles.
- Upright posture should be encouraged where equipment permits.
- Rowing is only appropriate for experienced participants who have regained lumbopelvic stability.
- The elliptical action of the cross-trainer is preferable to the stepper.
- Swimming is an excellent CV activity.
- Lumbopelvic stability is compromised after respiratory fatigue.

RESISTANCE TRAINING

10

BENEFITS OF RESISTANCE TRAINING

Increased strength and endurance, particularly in the upper body, is a necessity for postnatal women. The physical demands of lifting and carrying the baby and accompanying equipment suggest the need to develop upper body strength, and this can be achieved far more effectively with the use of resistance equipment. A programme that targets postural muscles, particularly those destabilised through pregnancy, and major muscles involved in lifting and carrying should be extremely beneficial in reducing the demands of everyday life and supporting weakened structures. In addition to the benefits of bone loading for increased bone density, recent studies by Lovelady et al. (2009) suggest that resistance training may actually slow down bone loss during lactation. Improved muscle mass as a result of resistance training also increases energy expenditure and assists with weight loss.

IMPLICATIONS

Joints and relaxin

Joint vulnerability is a key issue when training with weights and they should be introduced with caution to prevent injury. Correct posture and exercise technique is vital, together with the selection of low-risk exercises. The pelvis, in particular the SP and SIJ, needs particular care, and global muscles attaching into the pelvis should be trained carefully, e.g. gluteal group, hamstrings, adductors and hip flexors, as problems with reduced joint stability and alignment changes may only be revealed when weights are introduced. Previous PGP sufferers should be treated with extreme caution until the problem has completely resolved. *Women suffering from the continued effects of PGP should not be training with free weights.*

Lumbopelvic stability

Reduced lumbopelvic stability has implications for all exercise but is particularly crucial when adding an external resistance. *For this reason it is essential that the information in chapter 2 has been fully understood before training a postnatal client.* While the introduction of equipment may be appropriate for the muscles selected, reduced lumbopelvic stability does raise concerns for postural alignment. Delayed activation of the deep stabilisers will compromise all movements and increase the risk of injury.

The combined use of correct breathing techniques and retraining the brain to activate the deep stabilisers prior to movement is a vital routine to establish, and time should be spent explaining and learning this recruitment pattern. Adopting an upright position during seated or standing exercises should be encouraged wherever possible as this alignment switches on the inner unit. As soon as movement occurs, the global stabilisers (RA/EO/gluteus maximus) are activated to assist with support but account should be taken of their post-pregnancy reduction in strength. The greater the resistance used, the harder these muscles have to work to maintain support. Progression, therefore, should be dependent on the strength of the stabilisers rather than of the prime mover.

Overhead movements in particular, such as the lat pull-down, need careful observation to ensure that correct alignment is maintained – keeping the weights slightly forward and not lifting directly above the head will reduce the risk.

Abdominals

Getting into and out of position should be considered, as the weak, stretched abdominal musculature can easily be stressed by poor transitions. Equipment that requires the participant to be in a supine position, e.g. bench press, should be avoided if doming occurs in the abdominals when moving into place (*see* page 44). An imprinted spinal position (*see* page 40), with feet on the floor/bench, is safer to use when working with weights in a supine position: this allows a safer margin of error if alignment cannot be maintained. *Moving into and out of supine lying while holding the weights is inappropriate and unsafe.* Supine resisted exercises for RA and the obliques are contraindicated until the former has shortened and realigned – even then, the effectiveness of this type of exercise is questionable (*see* chapter 3)!

Pelvic floor muscles

These muscles have stretched and weakened during pregnancy and may have been further stressed by a vaginal delivery (*see* chapter 4). The PFM are part of the inner unit of muscles responsible for lumbopelvic stability and it is in this context that they are most at risk (*see* chapter 2). Lifting heavy weights without the support of the inner unit muscles will increase the stress to the PFM, which cannot resist the force of increased IAP (*see* figure 4.9, page 64).

Resistance training and dysfunctional PFM

O'Dwyer (2009) suggests that activities which increase the load on the PFM are completely inappropriate for women with dysfunctional PFM. With this in mind, if 50 per cent of postnatal women have some degree of pelvic organ prolapse (Hagen et al. 2006) instructors should question the suitability of resistance training for their clients at this time!

Over-recruitment of RA and EO, in an attempt to provide sufficient stability, will have a similar effect on the PFM as will breath holding and the use of the Valsalva manoeuvre (*see* below). A good indication of loss of support from the inner unit is when the abdomen pushes out, as this suggests that the PFM are also being pushed downwards. Close observation is essential.

Breasts

Hormonal changes with breastfeeding will prolong the effects of joint laxity and compromise muscular strength (*see* chapter 5). Breastfeeding may also reduce the choice of equipment available: the selection of appropriate exercises should have regard to the increased size and the comfort of the breasts, which may feel tender if squeezed or bumped. This will apply to the seated pec dec, any prone lying exercises, and all seated exercises with chest pads (preacher curl, seated row etc.). Body positioning and joint alignment should not be compromised in order to perform such exercises comfortably; this particularly applies to prone lying, where placing the hands under the breasts to reduce the pressure may increase lumbar lordosis. A forwards leaning position, such as four-point kneeling, may cause additional drag and discomfort to heavy breasts. Free weights usage may necessitate slight adaptations to work within a comfortable range of movement, e.g. biceps curl adapted to hammer curl, to avoid bumping the breasts with a bulky dumbbell. Consideration should also be given to the possible leakage of milk if an excessive amount of arm work is performed; body parts should be worked in rotation and repetitions closely monitored.

Forearm, wrist and hand pain

Problems in these areas will have implications for holding resistance equipment and this will prevent sufferers from participating in upper body work (*see* chapter 6). The following points should be considered for women recovering from these conditions:

- Flexion of the supporting wrists during weight-bearing exercises (triceps kickback, single-arm row, press-up) may cause tingling and numbness in the thumb and first two fingers.
- Poor wrist/forearm alignment in any position may cause discomfort. Exercises using resistance bands need particularly close observation.
- Wrapping a resistance band around the fingers will restrict blood flow.
- Grip strength may be affected.
- Thumb adduction – necessary for holding the weights – may be painful.

Correct wrist alignment must be observed at all times and over-gripping discouraged. Tingling or numbness is less likely to occur when the hands are in an elevated position.

CONSIDERATIONS

Strength or endurance?

Strength training should be avoided until joint and lumbopelvic stability has been gained. Working to failure will be detrimental to the joints and stabilising muscles, and may compromise spinal safety. Endurance work is recommended, using a high repetition range and low resistance.

What is the Valsalva manoeuvre?

This is a condition associated with strength training when additional trunk support is needed for the maximum application of force. It may also occur with coughing or straining on the toilet. The breath is held and pressure in the thoracic cavity increases as air is prevented from escaping. This coping strategy may also be adopted with endurance training when the resistance is just a little too much to be able to continue to the end of a set of repetitions. As the muscles struggle to cope the breath is held, blood pressure and IAP rise, and pressure is exerted on the abdominal and pelvic floor muscles. Selection of the appropriate number of sets and repetitions for the individual is essential. Excessive training may encourage breath holding as fatigue sets in.

Closed and open chain exercises

This refers to the linking system of the body made by a series of joints that connect bones to one another.

A closed chain exercise relates to the working limb or limbs being fixed to an external resistance, e.g. floor or stable piece of equipment, so that the joints move in a predetermined way! It requires multiple joint and muscle actions to occur at once, which is mostly how the body functions in ADL. Closed chain exercises are more suitable than open chain exercises for postnatal women as the compressive forces exerted through the joints help with stability. Closed chain exercises enhance proprioception, and feedback is provided by the stability of the lever. Examples are: fixed resistance equipment, the Pilates Reformer, some exercises using a resistance band, e.g. when it is secured under the feet in sitting or standing, and press-ups.

An open chain exercise is when the working limb or limbs are not attached to anything at the end and are free to move in any direction. It can target specific muscles, which is beneficial for rehabilitation; however, joint risk increases with the addition of a weight onto the end of the lever. The knees in particular are vulnerable to injury from open chain exercises such as leg curl and leg extension. Resistance training using free weights is mostly open chain and needs careful instruction and observation to reduce the risk of injury.

Free weights v fixed resistance equipment

Fixed resistance equipment cannot always replicate joint action and some of the positions may not be comfortable for postnatal women. On some older equipment where the range of movement is not adjustable there is an increased risk of hyperextension, e.g. of the shoulder and lumbar spine, and sometimes the minimum resistance available may still be too heavy for some women.

Fixed resistance equipment does, however, provide a stable body position and most exercises are closed chain. The preset range of movement previously mentioned can be advantageous, preventing overextension of joints, although range adjusters are available with the majority of equipment. Much less skill is required to use fixed resistance equipment and it would seem to be a very appropriate method of training for an inexperienced person, provided a comprehensive induction has been given.

Free weights, body bars, weighted balls, resistance bands etc. are beneficial as they can replicate the action of the joint in a variety of body positions. They all, however, require good lumbopelvic stability to support the spine and are often open chain. The heavier the resistance, the greater the demand on the stabilising muscles and this should be considered when progressing the exercises, even if the prime mover is coping adequately. The use of light equipment is recommended once lumbopelvic stability has been gained – close observation of technique is vital.

Kettlebell training

This activity is contraindicated for postnatal women. A dynamic, open chain activity involving a swinging weight on destabilised joints with poor lumbopelvic stability and possible PFM dysfunction – kettlebell training is a recipe for disaster! Participation should be postponed until joint and lumbopelvic stability has been regained, breastfeeding stopped and strength improved by more suitable whole-body workouts.

Vibration training

Vibration training may initially sound ideal for postnatal women. As a low-impact, low-loading activity, some of the potential benefits are claimed to be improved circulation, increased muscle activity, improved bone density, decreased blood pressure, and weight loss. However, in the absence of specific research relating to vibration training for postnatal women, this activity should be approached with caution. Training should be supervised at all times by a qualified vibration training instructor and the session adapted to the needs of the individual. Women should not be left to their own devices on this equipment! The following considerations relate to structural changes that may be magnified by this type of training:

- Reduced joint stability
- Poor postural alignment
- Reduced lumbopelvic stability
- Increased pressure on the PFM

Vibration training is inappropriate for breast-feeding mums!

Position selection

Some fixed resistance equipment may be unsuitable due to body position. All seated exercises with chest pads (preacher curl, seated row etc.) may feel extremely uncomfortable for women who are breastfeeding, as will prone positions discussed earlier. The latter may also be inappropriate for women who delivered by caesarean section due to the possible discomfort experienced around the site of the scar. The supine position itself is appropriate but the transition into it may stress the abdominals and increase separation of the two muscular bands. Side lying, before rolling over onto the back, is recommended for floorwork, but is not possible on a bench! Many exercises using an external resistance, such as bands and free weights, can be performed standing or sitting.

Range of movement

In order to work effectively, joints should be taken through their full range of movement, although particular care must be taken to prevent overextending, which will increase the risk of injury to vulnerable joints. All seated fixed resistance equipment needs careful adjustment to ensure that joints are working within a correct range of movement. *The 'total hip'*

machine, still going in some gyms, is not suitable for postnatal women due to its poor design and frequent misuse!

How soon can training begin?

Following a satisfactory postnatal check-up, a programme of lumbopelvic retraining should be commenced. All participants, experienced or not, must establish good inner unit activation and co-ordination before weights are introduced (*see* chapter 2). Movement patterns should be rehearsed without resistance at first as this will retrain the brain to activate the inner unit for each particular movement pattern. Once this has been achieved and the four deep stabilisers can be activated in co-ordination, the load can be gradually increased.

This introductory level may be difficult for experienced participants, who may wish to return to the gym immediately and recommence where they left off! *Education and encouragement is essential.*

What are the intensity recommendations for experienced clients?

Assuming the above has been adhered to, experienced clients are advised to work at 70 per cent of the weight they used prior to pregnancy. This may gradually increase, over a period of weeks, to the pre-pregnancy resistance, but the emphasis should remain on endurance training until joint stability has returned. In addition to the workload on the stabilising muscles, intensity considerations should also relate to breastfeeding: moderate-intensity training and good hydration is recommended to maintain milk quality and quantity. Training to failure should *not* resume until breastfeeding has ceased and joint stability returned.

And if the client is inexperienced?

Again, assuming the earlier recommendations have been adhered to, newcomers to weights should begin with the lightest weight available. This practice run provides better feedback than a weight-free rehearsal. The resistance selected for the main workout should be sufficient to bring on mild fatigue on the last repetition of a 12–20 repetition set. Correct breathing must be practised to avoid the risk of breath holding and the possible triggering of the Valsalva manoeuvre. Joint alignment and exercise technique is absolutely vital at this time. The newcomer needs careful guidance from an instructor on transitions into and out of machines, handling free weights, and the exercise itself. Close observation and correction is expected.

Target muscle groups

The selection of appropriate muscles will depend on individual postural changes, but the aims are to strengthen muscles that have been lengthened and weakened by pregnancy postural changes, e.g. gluteus maximus, lower trapezius, posterior rotator cuff. Inner range training (*see* page 26) should be included where appropriate. Consideration should also be given to muscles required to support vulnerable joints, e.g. gluteus medius/minimus and vastus medialis, as well as those muscles involved in lifting and carrying, e.g. latissimus dorsi, biceps, triceps and quadriceps.

Are there any exercises that should be avoided?

The introduction of exercises for the adductor group muscles should be treated with caution due to the vulnerability of SP and possible stress to the joint when the muscles are contracted. Exercises for the abductor muscles may also cause problems for SP or SIJ. See chapter 6 for guidelines for these exercises in PGP sufferers. Exercises or transitions which cause the abdominals to dome should be eliminated until appropriate recovery is made. Any exercise performed with incorrect technique should be stopped immediately. The suitability of the shoulder press and pec dec should be considered in relation to target muscles and postnatal posture: upper trapezius and pectorals may already be tight, particularly if the shoulders are protracted. The chest press is a more suitable choice. The upright row should be modified to assist with lifting and carrying, and range of movement reduced to avoid training the upper trapezius. Studio resistance training is discussed in chapter 12.

Guidelines for a resistance training session

- Select appropriate exercises for the target muscle groups.
- Consider position and range of movement.
- Rehearse the movement pattern, focusing on recruitment of the deep stabilising muscles.
- Select an appropriate weight to experience mild fatigue on the last repetition.
- Assume correct starting position, with good postural alignment and neutral spine.
- Consciously activate TrA and the PFM prior to doing the first repetition.
- Complete 12–20 repetitions in one set.
- Observe strict adherence to correct technique.
- Perform each repetition slowly and with control.
- Rest and repeat – a further set may be performed after a short break of approximately 45 seconds, or later in the workout.
- Exercise body parts in rotation – one upper body exercise followed by one lower body exercise to prevent early fatigue.

Table 10.1	Additional considerations for the use of fixed resistance machines (cont.)
Adductor press	Getting into position
	PGP sufferers
	Lumbopelvic stability
	Back hyperextension
	Overly large ROM
	NB: Perform both legs together.
	Ensure that ROM is adjusted to suit the individual.

SELECTED EXERCISES USING PORTABLE RESISTANCE EQUIPMENT

The following exercises are intended for use once lumbopelvic stability has been restored. For variety, two types of resistance have been selected – bands and dumbbells – as these are the most readily available, practical pieces of equipment. Some of the exercises can be performed with other equipment, while others are only suitable for one type of resistance.

Figure 10.1 Rotator cuff

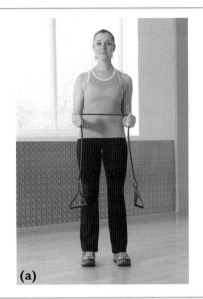
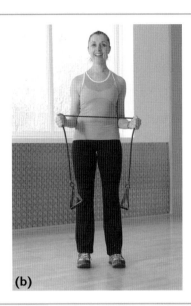

(a) (b)

Resistance band

Rotator cuff

Purpose: to strengthen the muscles of the posterior shoulder and draw the humerus back into its correct position. External rotation is more beneficial for kyphotic changes.

Preparation

Stand in correct upright posture, with feet hip-width apart and spine in neutral. Hold a resistance band in front at waist height, with palms facing in, thumbs on top and wrists/forearms aligned. Band should be straight but not taut. Draw elbows into the waist and lengthen the shoulders and ribcage downwards.

Action

Inhale to prepare and as you exhale recruit TrA and open the shoulders to the sides, keeping elbows tight into waistline, pulling the resistance band outwards. Release and return with control. Maintain natural breathing throughout.

Technique tips

- Maintain correct postural alignment throughout – do not lean back as the arms open.
- Use the abdominals to draw the ribcage down.
- Slide the shoulder blades down as the arms open.
- Maintain wrist and forearm alignment.

Progression

Use a stronger resistance band to intensify the exercise.

Caution: Wrapping the band around the hands will restrict blood flow and should be avoided.

Figure 10.2 Trapezius squeeze

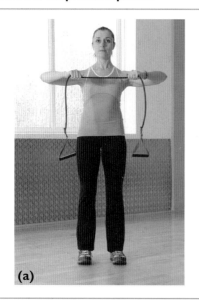

(a)

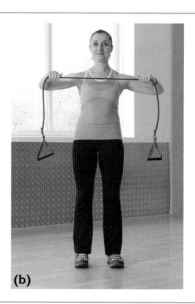

(b)

Trapezius squeeze

Purpose: to strengthen the mid-trapezius and rhomboid muscles in their inner range to reduce muscle length and improve posture.

Preparation

Stand in correct upright posture, with feet hip-width apart and spine in neutral. Hold a resistance band in front at chest height. Lift the elbows and keep wrists/forearms aligned. Lengthen the shoulders and ribcage downwards.

Action

Inhale to prepare and while exhaling recruit TrA and pull the band apart, drawing the shoulder blades downwards and inwards. Release with control. Maintain natural breathing.

Technique tips

- Maintain correct postural alignment throughout – do not lean back as the arms open.
- Use the abdominals to draw the ribcage down.
- Maintain wrist and forearm alignment.
- Keep the elbows lifted.
- Draw the shoulder blades down as the arms open.

Progression

Double the band up to increase the resistance before moving to a stronger band.

Figure 10.3 Seated row

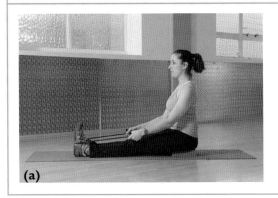
(a)

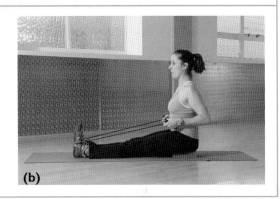
(b)

Seated row

Purpose: to strengthen the mid-trapezius, latissimus dorsi and biceps to assist postural correction and lifting/carrying.

Preparation

Sit on a block on the floor, with legs extended in front, knees slightly bent. Lengthen the spine and lift out of your sit bones – you may need to bend the knees a little more for comfort. Wrap a resistance band around the soles of the feet and hold each end with thumbs on top, arms reaching forwards. Lengthen the shoulder blades and ribcage downwards.

Action

Inhale to prepare and as you exhale recruit TrA and draw the arms back, leading with the elbows and bending them in close to the body. Keep the back in an upright position. Return to starting position, keeping the upper back lifted. Maintain natural breathing.

Technique tips

- Maintain correct postural alignment throughout.
- Avoid arching the back as the arms draw back.
- Avoid bending forwards on return.
- Keep lifted on sit bones – don't rock back.
- Use the abdominals to draw the ribcage down.
- Keep the shoulder blades drawing down throughout.
- Maintain wrist and forearm alignment.
- Keep the elbows close to the body.
- Bend the knees further if the hamstrings are pulling.

Progression

Use a stronger resistance band to intensify the exercise.

Figure 10.4 Chest press

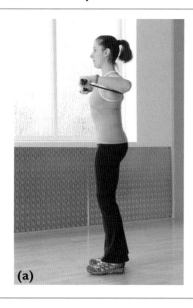

(a)

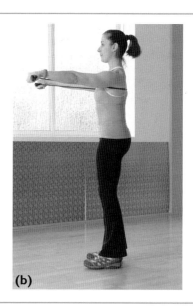

(b)

Chest press

Purpose: to strengthen the pectorals to increase breast support and assist with lifting and carrying.

Preparation

Stand in correct upright posture, with feet hip-width apart and spine in neutral. Wrap a resistance band around your back and under your armpits, and hold the ends, with arms bent at shoulder height, palms to the floor. Relax your shoulders and ensure that wrists and forearms are aligned.

Action

Inhale to prepare and as you exhale recruit TrA and push the arms forwards in line with the shoulders. Keep the elbows slightly bent, wrist/forearms aligned and shoulders down. Return to starting position. Maintain natural breathing.

Technique tips

- Maintain correct postural alignment throughout.
- Avoid leaning back onto the band as the arms straighten.
- Avoid hyperextending the spine as the arms release.
- Keep the arms shoulder-width apart.
- Use the abdominals to draw the ribcage down.
- Keep the shoulder blades drawing down throughout.
- Maintain wrist and forearm alignment.

Alternative

This exercise can also be performed lying supine pushing dumbbells or body bar to the ceiling.

Figure 10.5 Pull-down

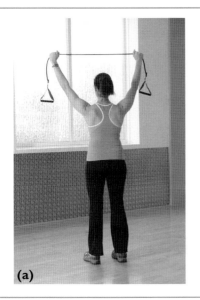
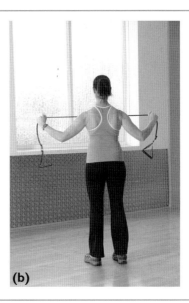

(a)

(b)

Pull-down

Purpose: to strengthen the lower trapezius and latissimus dorsi muscles to help reduce postural kyphosis.

Preparation

Stand in correct upright posture, with feet hip-width apart and spine in neutral. With an over-hand grip, hold a resistance band in front, arms shoulder-width apart. Lift the arms up diagonally in front of the head, keeping the elbows soft. Keep the body weight centred, check neutral again and slide the shoulder blades down.

Action

Inhale to prepare and as you exhale recruit TrA and pull the band outwards and downwards so the central point of the band moves towards the breastbone and the elbows bend in towards the waist. Slowly return to the starting position, focusing on drawing the tips of the shoulder blades down towards the hips. Maintain natural breathing.

Technique tips

- Maintain correct postural alignment throughout.
- Avoid leaning back as the arms lower.
- Make a semi-circular shape with the arms on both phases.
- Keep the shoulder blades drawing down.
- Use the abdominals to draw the ribcage down.
- Maintain wrist/forearm alignment.
- Focus on the upward phase of movement.

Progression

Pull down on one side only, keeping the other arm in the lifted position. This increases the load on the stabilising muscles to maintain balance and control.

Figure 10.6 Biceps curl

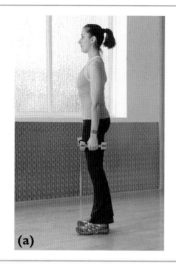

(a)

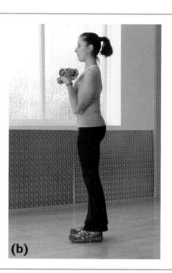

(b)

Dumbbells

Biceps curl

Purpose: to strengthen the biceps to assist with lifting and carrying.

Preparation

Stand in correct upright posture, with feet hip-width apart and spine in neutral. Hold a dumbbell in each hand with arms relaxed by sides and palms facing inwards. Check the wrists and forearms are aligned and slide the shoulder blades down. Soften the knees.

Action

Inhale to prepare and as you exhale recruit TrA and curl the lower arms up towards the shoulders, rotating the forearms as you lift so that the palms face the shoulders. Lower the arms with control, rotating the forearms back so the palms face inwards. Straighten the elbows but do not lock out. Maintain natural breathing.

Technique tips

- Stand tall, maintaining correct postural alignment throughout.
- Draw the ribcage down as the arms lift to avoid leaning back.
- Keep the elbows tucked into the sides.
- Avoid locking out the elbows as they lower.
- Keep the shoulder blades drawing down throughout.
- Maintain wrist and forearm alignment.
- Avoid over-gripping the dumbbell.
- Perform slowly with control.

Alternative

This exercise can be performed seated on a chair/bench or kneeling. Alternatively, fix a resistance band under both feet at hip-width apart, or under one foot in split stance if the band is short. Hold around each end of the band with thumbs on top, forearms parallel to the floor. If this is too intense, work one arm at a time so the band is longer.

Figure 10.7 Modified upright row

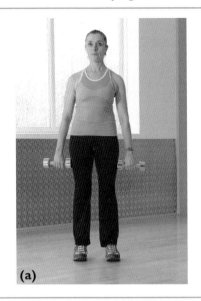
(a)

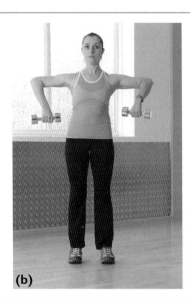
(b)

Modified upright row

Purpose: to strengthen the biceps and deltoids to assist with lifting and carrying.

Preparation

Stand in correct upright posture, with feet hip-width apart and spine in neutral. Hold a dumbbell in each hand with an overhand grip, palms facing back and arms shoulder-width apart. Check the wrists and forearms are aligned and slide the shoulder blades down. Soften the knees.

Action

Inhale to prepare and while exhaling recruit TrA and lift the arms up, bending the elbows out to the sides until hands are on a level with the lower ribcage. Do not lift any higher as this will activate the upper trapezius, which may already be tight from postural changes. Lower slowly until the arms are straight but not locked. Maintain natural breathing.

Technique tips

- Stand tall and maintain correct postural alignment throughout.
- Draw the ribcage down as the arms lift, to avoid leaning back.
- Keep the shoulder blades sliding down.
- Maintain wrist and forearm alignment as the arms lift.
- Avoid over-gripping the dumbbell.
- Perform slowly and with control.

Alternative

In the same position, but with a resistance band under both feet.

Figure 10.8 Dumbbell squat

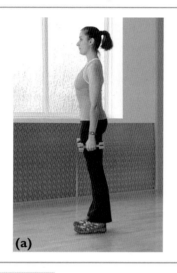

(a)

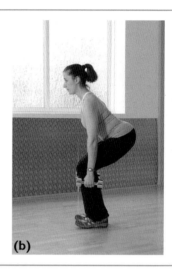

(b)

Dumbbell squat

Purpose: to strengthen the gluteals, hamstrings and quadriceps to assist with lumbopelvic stability, postural realignment and lifting.

Preparation

Stand in correct upright posture, with feet hip-width apart and spine in neutral. Hold a dumb-bell in each hand, with palms facing inwards and arms relaxed by sides. Slide the shoulder blades down and stand tall.

Action

Inhale to prepare and as you exhale recruit TrA and bend the knees, hinging at the hips but maintaining neutral spine. Allow the arms to fall naturally towards the knees. Do not bend below 90 degrees. Return to the upright position without locking out the knees. Maintain natural breathing.

Technique tips

- Maintain correct postural alignment throughout.
- Ensure that the abdominals are activated prior to the first repetition.
- Take the body weight back towards the heels.
- Lengthen the spine away from the floor as you lower.
- Let the weight of the dumbbells draw the shoulders down.
- Keep looking straight ahead – avoid looking down.
- Keep knees aligned in parallel.
- Imagine you're lowering yourself onto a chair.
- Fully extend the knees and hips as you return.
- Perform slowly with control.
- Practise first without the dumbbells.

Caution: The back is at risk with this exercise if the deep stabilisers cannot be recruited.

GROUP FITNESS SESSIONS

11

This chapter looks at different types of exercise session and discusses their suitability for post-natal women. *As with any activity, the suitability of the session is dependent on the underpinning knowledge and expertise of the instructor.*

SPECIFIC POSTNATAL EXERCISE CLASS

Suitability

This is obviously the ideal – *assuming the instructor is qualified to teach this specialist group!* Attendance can commence following a satisfactory postnatal check-up or 8–10 weeks following a caesarean section. While this type of class will probably attract the less-fit or previously inexperienced mum, the regular exerciser also needs to return to basics to retrain lumbopelvic stability and restore postural alignment. The additional social benefits of a specific postnatal class are invaluable to all new mums. Regardless of the length of time that has elapsed since delivery, a carefully structured educational programme is an excellent introduction to exercise at any time.

Considerations

Specific postnatal exercise sessions should consider all the implications of pregnancy and delivery, and the effects of breastfeeding, continued joint instability, reduced lumbopelvic stability and postural change. Movements should be simple and easy to follow, and concentrate on working weakened muscles and stretching tightened ones to redress pregnancy changes. A great deal of emphasis should be placed on retraining lumbopelvic stability and correcting poor postural alignment. All exercises should be suitable and provision made for alternative positions and/or exercises where appropriate.

The social and emotional benefits of a specific postnatal exercise session are invaluable. It provides an opportunity to meet other new mums and to share the concerns and anxieties of early motherhood. It is also a non-threatening exercise environment, with the majority of women concerned about lack of muscular tone in their abdomen and the struggle to lose extra weight gained during pregnancy.

BUGGY WORKOUT

Suitability

Since this is also a specific postnatal exercise session, it is vital that instructors hold a specialist postnatal qualification. Just because the class is conducted outside and mums are involved in walking activities does not mean that the instructor is exempt from such a qualification. If anything, it requires a much higher level of teaching and expertise than an indoor session (*see* Useful Contacts for details of Pushy Mothers instructor training courses).

An outdoor buggy workout offers fresh air, vitamin D for mother and baby, and no childcare concerns or special equipment. Subject to a satisfactory postnatal check-up it is suitable for all new mums from 10 weeks onwards and will attract all types – particularly those unaccustomed to regular exercise, who may feel more comfortable in this environment.

Considerations

An appropriately structured session should address all relevant postnatal issues as discussed above. Running with the buggy and exercising while holding the baby are contraindicated and should not be included in any exercise session (*see* chapter 9). Fast turning movements with the buggy may compromise the wrist, and pushing up hill should be closely observed to ensure good postural alignment (*see* page 178).

BOOT CAMPS

Suitability

Outdoor fitness is enjoying a surge in popularity and fitness boot camps are appearing in parks all over the country. Content varies but the general theme is a full-on, sixty-minute workout, combining interspersed circuit training moves (curl-ups, star jumps, burpees, press-ups etc.) with running and team games in a competitive, fun session that is all-inclusive. *This kind of workout is unsuitable for postnatal women until joint and lumbopelvic stability has been regained, breastfeeding ceased and fitness improved in a more controlled setting.*

PILATES

Suitability

Pilates may seem ideal for postnatal women: its slow, controlled movements with emphasis on correct joint alignment are designed to improve posture by appropriate selection of strengthening and stretching exercises. Appropriate Pilates exercises are included in chapter 3.

Suitability of Pilates

Specific postnatal Pilates classes taught by a qualified postnatal Pilates instructor are recommended but mainstream classes raise many more concerns. A good percentage of 'popular' Pilates movements involve resisted trunk flexion and this action is unsuitable for the majority of postnatal women until lumbopelvic stability has been restored (see chapter 3). It is likely to exacerbate incorrect muscle patterns and increases the risk of prolapse.

Considerations

All postnatal women, with or without previous experience of Pilates, should start with the basic principles before progressing too quickly. Learning to recruit TrA correctly without gripping and holding is difficult for any newcomer to Pilates, but a postnatal newcomer has the additional disadvantages of a weakened inner unit with possible faulty timing mechanisms (*see* chapter 2).

Selection of appropriate low-risk exercises and inclusion of functional training are essential. Prone positions may be uncomfortable for breastfeeding women and adaptations may be necessary. Exercises which encourage RA lengthening are inappropriate. All exercises should commence with a cue for TrA recruitment but no further reminders should be given until the particular exercise has been completed. Constant cueing to draw in TrA will encourage over-recruitment of the global stabilisers (*see* chapter 2).

YOGA

Suitability

As discussed for Pilates, yoga is only suitable if the instructor has a specialist postnatal yoga qualification, or mums attend a specific postnatal yoga class. With appropriate guidance and good instruction this can be very beneficial in improving posture, aiding digestion, releasing muscular tension and aiding relaxation.

All yoga styles are descendants of the original Hatha yoga, which encompasses mind, body and spirit. It is the easiest, most relaxing of styles and is the most suitable for postnatal women. Iyengar yoga is stricter than Hatha and involves holding poses for longer, which may be too demanding; Ashtanga is an advanced form requiring strength, stamina and flexibility.

Considerations

The main concerns relate to range of movement and joint alignment. Pushing the body beyond its natural range is contraindicated at this time and modifications should be offered wherever appropriate. Prone positions may be uncomfortable for breastfeeding mums and movements such as the 'Bow' are contraindicated. A modified 'Cobra' should be included to reduce range of movement and avoid stretching RA – this position is beneficial for opening the chest. Pelvic rotational movements may stress the SIJ and wide-standing postures may cause discomfort to the SP. Changes in femur alignment may trigger knee and pelvic discomfort in the 'Warrior' pose, although this posture is particularly good for stretching tight hip flexors. The 'Lotus' should be avoided until knee stability has been regained. Excellent for lengthening spinal extensors, the 'Downward-Facing Dog' is performed with heels up and knees bent, although the breasts may drag uncomfortably in this position. An inverted position should be avoided in the early weeks and reintroduced with modifications. This position may be beneficial for aiding venous return and reducing swelling and can be very helpful for re-educating the PFM.

STRETCH CLASS

Suitability

Stretching can be extremely beneficial in reducing muscular tension, and the selection of appropriate stretches will help to improve poor posture. The calm, controlled nature of a stretch class may also help to reduce emotional stress and encourage the body to rest and relax.

Considerations

While stretching to *maintain* flexibility is valuable and recommended, stretching to improve flexibility should be avoided in the first few months after delivery, longer if breastfeeding (*see* chapter 1). Connective tissue changes, as a result of increased relaxin production, allow a greater range of joint movement and this may result in overstretching of the ligaments. Joint alignment should be considered in all stretch positions to ensure that safety is not compromised. Adductor stretches should be approached with caution for women who have recovered from PGP as these muscles are likely to feel extremely tight.

Some seated floor positions may be uncomfortable for the perineum, and prone lying uncomfortable for breastfeeding mums. Stretches for the abdominal muscles are inappropriate at this time – the emphasis of postnatal abdominal recovery is on shortening and realigning the muscles. Those who had a caesarean delivery may experience discomfort with stretches that pull on the abdomen, e.g. gluteal stretch and lying body stretch.

BODY CONDITIONING CLASS

Suitability

This encompasses a variety of class types, often with quirky names, but usually relating to muscular endurance training without a CV component. It is a popular choice for new mums as it often includes exercises for abdominal muscles, which many women believe will give them a flat tummy (*see* chapter 3)! The absence of high-impact work is also attractive – breast discomfort and the fear of leaking being their main concerns. Such classes often include the use of small equipment such as hand weights and resistance bands.

Considerations

As always, joint alignment and range of movement are important in avoiding joint stress. These concerns, together with reduced lumbopelvic stability, are particularly crucial if resistance equipment is used (*see* chapter 10). Pelvic and abdominal care is required during position transitions, and women recovering from PGP should be shown how to move correctly; exercises for the abductors and/or adductors may cause discomfort for these women (*see* chapter 6). Abdominal work should focus on correct recruitment of TrA and progress according to the guidelines given in chapter 3. Resisted flexion should be avoided and the focus changed to recruiting the abdominal muscles in a more functional way – i.e. standing exercises.

Prone floor positions will probably be uncomfortable if breastfeeding. Some of the exercises can be adapted to a box position on elbows and knees, while others will need alternative exercises. Seated floor positions may be uncomfortable for the perineum and may also require a change of position.

HIGH/LOW AEROBIC CLASSES

Suitability of high/low aerobic classes

High-impact aerobics is inappropriate for postnatal mums because of increased stress to the joints, breasts and in particular PFM (see chapter 4). Likewise, a fast-paced low-impact class with motivating music and ineffective teaching will also be inappropriate! While low-impact moves should be much safer and can be equally effective, it is down to the choice of movements, speed, execution and instructor expertise.

Considerations

Movements that stress the joints do not necessarily involve jumping; some seemingly low-impact moves can still create an increased degree of stress purely through poor performance. Marching on the spot, for example, if performed with a heavy downward stamp can create a similar amount of force to that of jumping. Keeping the body lifted and emphasising the upward movement of the legs will reduce the impact considerably. Fast knee-bending movements increase the impact on the PFM and may feel most uncomfortable. Such movements should be performed at half speed or an alternative exercise provided. Correct joint alignment should be closely monitored and particular care taken to avoid excessive pelvic movement. Women recovering from PGP may need to reduce the width of sidesteps and all movements performed on one leg should maintain a lift through the supporting hip.

Varied use of directions is particularly helpful for improving bone density but directional changes should be choreographed into the routine and appropriately cued to allow time for the transition (*see* chapter 5). Rapid changes of direction are unsuitable and increase the risk of ankle and knee injury.

Correct upright posture should be encouraged throughout, as this aids recruitment of the deep stabilising muscles (*see* chapter 2). Use of forward arm movements may encourage rounding in the upper body, particularly if the breasts are heavy, and when the arms are taken behind the body or above the head, the back is more likely to hyperextend. Reducing the range of backward arm movements and keeping the arms further forwards when working above the head will help to maintain correct spinal alignment. Drawing the ribcage down will assist correction.

Excessive use of wide-range arm movements or crossing in front of the chest, particularly with momentum, may cause the breasts to leak. Exercise intensity should be kept to a moderate level, with good hydration to maintain milk quality and quantity. A supportive bra (or two) is essential to reduce breast movement and minimise bounce

– breast pads may also be necessary. Appropriate, supportive footwear is vital to provide adequate shock absorption and increased ankle stability.

DANCE-BASED WORKOUTS

Suitability

This is an umbrella term for a variety of dance styles – some more appropriate than others for postnatal women. These sessions will improve co-ordination, agility and cardiovascular fitness, and burn unwanted calories – they can also be great fun! The rise in popularity of Latin American style dance classes presents a few concerns relating to pelvic stability, as does belly dancing. Pole dancing also involves pelvic movements and performing on the pole will be very uncomfortable for breastfeeding mums! Tap dancing is not suitable for breastfeeding mums and reduced ankle stability increases the risk of injury.

Considerations

Participation in dance styles that encourage excessive pelvic movement should be delayed until joint and lumbopelvic stability has been regained. Some dance styles, such as salsa, are particularly beneficial for increasing thoracic mobility and may be an appropriate choice after regaining the stability. Women recovering from PGP should be cautious. As with many activities, music and atmosphere increase the risks, as the mood takes over and technical performance decreases. Breasts may need additional support for this type of activity.

STEP CLASS

Suitability

This cardiovascular activity can be a valuable form of exercise *if undertaken at an appropriate level*. Simple, easy to follow step patterns may be a far more beneficial workout for the inexperienced exerciser than attempting to follow the co-ordinated movements of an aerobics class. Directional changes also help to improve bone density by loading the bone in a variety of ways.

There are concerns, however, relating to the continuous, repetitive nature of the activity, particularly if posture is poor. Correct ankle and knee alignment is essential to avoid additional stress to joints still lacking stability from connective tissue changes. Women with everted ankles should be discouraged from participating. The speed and complexity of the class, together with the ability of the instructor to provide alternative exercises, are most significant in determining suitability for attendance. *Step is not suitable for women recovering from PGP.*

Considerations

The stepping action should be reviewed to ensure that the whole foot is correctly placed on the step every time and that the ankles are supported to prevent rolling. When stepping up, the knees should straighten but not lock out and the pelvis should remain in a neutral position. The spine is particularly vulnerable, especially when lifting the leg behind, with a natural tendency to arch the back; upper body weight should be adjusted forwards and the ribcage drawn down to prevent this occurring. Step height should be considered in relation to the degree of lateral pelvic rocking: excessive movement may stress the SP/SIJ and should be avoided. Side leg raises should be kept low and care taken not to tip or twist the pelvis. The ballistic nature of power moves will increase stress to the joints, PFM and breasts. Correct upright posture must be maintained throughout to activate the deep stabilising muscles, and appropriate support is needed to minimise movement of the breasts.

WATER WORKOUTS

12

BENEFITS OF POSTNATAL WATER WORKOUTS

- **Reduced joint stress:** One of the major benefits of water workouts is the reduction in the amount of stress to weight-bearing joints. Structures destabilised during pregnancy, through connective tissue changes and increased weight gain, are supported by the water when submerged.
- **Increased circulation:** The pressure of water exerted on the blood vessels stimulates the circulation and increases the stroke volume (amount of blood pumped on each cardiac contraction). This induces a lower working heart rate than on land. Improved circulation also helps relieve constipation.
- **Increased venous return:** Water pressure encourages a more effective return of blood and prevents blood pooling in the legs. This is helpful for improving the condition of varicose veins.
- **Increased urinary output:** Increased circulation improves blood flow to the kidneys and increases urinary output. This helps with the loss of excess fluid retained during pregnancy.
- **Reduced swelling:** Hydrostatic pressure forces retained fluids out of the tissues into the circulation. This is particularly helpful for pelvic floor repair.
- **Reduced muscle soreness:** Exercising in water predominantly consists of concentric muscle work (this principle changes when flotation equipment is used). Muscular soreness is generally produced by eccentric work,

therefore the after-effects of a water workout are felt less than on land.
- **Soothing and calming effects:** Water can be very therapeutic in aiding postnatal recovery. The slower actions of the body and the massaging effects of the water induce a feeling of composure and relaxation. This often continues after the workout has finished.

IMPLICATIONS

Joints

Effects of gravity on the body are reduced by 80 per cent when immersed at chest depth. This cushioning allows the joints a greater ROM but because the resistance of the water slows movements down, the risk of injury from this increased ROM is reduced. Immersion to the waist reduces the effects of gravity by only 50 per cent: this has implications for joint and breast stress when jumping or if large-range upper body movements are performed.

Abdominals

The abdominal muscles play a key role in lumbopelvic stability (*see* chapter 2). As one of the local stabilisers, TrA works at very low levels to maintain control of spinal movements but in water, where the workload is greater, the global stabilisers (EO/IO) and even mobilisers (RA) are also required to help out. The deeper the water, the greater the workload. As the body becomes more buoyant these larger muscles must stabilise the torso to allow the arms and legs to move without the body moving in the opposite direction. In group sessions the workload on the abdominals intensifies with increased turbulence. While this is an effective way of working these muscles, care should be taken not to overdo it initially – working in shallower water and adopting a split stance for static movements will reduce the intensity of the workload on the abdominals. Upright postural alignment in the water will assist activation of the local stabilising muscles and this will ensure that the abdominals are working together to stabilise the linea alba. Movements that require strong trunk rotation should not be performed if the abdominals have a separation of more than two fingers (*see* chapter 3).

Pelvic floor

Due to the buoyancy of the body in water, risk to the pelvic floor is significantly reduced. Reduced gravitational pull makes it easier to engage the PFM so if an individual is experiencing difficulty with this exercise on land it may be a good alternative. The pressure of the water on the perineum will help to reduce any lingering swelling around the episiotomy or tear site by dispersing retained fluids and speeding up the healing process. Exercising in water increases urinary output and this may necessitate more frequent trips to the toilet.

Breasts

Breasts must be supported during water workouts of any type to prevent sagging and overstretching. Many swimsuits do not have the additional support of a shelf bra sewn into the garment: this could result in heavy breasts being supported by just one layer of very stretched fabric. It may be necessary to wear a bra under the swimsuit to reduce bounce. If the breasts remain immersed under the water there is less risk, but if they are above the water level the delicate breast tissue is just as vulnerable as during land-based exercise. Even with appropriate support, the drag effect of the water on the breasts when jumping can be extremely uncomfortable. When exercising in waist-deep water a wide leg base should be adopted with bent knees; not only does this keep the breasts immersed but it also provides greater stability and a more effective workout for the arms.

Feeding before exercising is always recommended but this may not prevent a loss of milk if vigorous large-range arm work is continued. Exercising in very warm water may encourage milk flow.

CONSIDERATIONS

Water resistance

The resistance of water is 12 times greater than that of air, and when the body is immersed the resistance is present in all directions of movement. The bigger the surface area, the greater the resistance, so standing in an upright position and walking through water is more intense than the horizontal swimming position. Group exercise sessions create turbulence, which further increases water resistance and can make it a very demanding activity. The intensity of the workload is determined by the amount of effort used – the greater the effort, the higher the workload. Speed increases the intensity so fast movements cannot be continued for very long and should be interspersed with slow sections. Interval training is particularly useful when returning to exercise, as the more demanding sections can be of short duration in the initial sessions, with the majority of the workout pitched at a moderate intensity.

Pool temperature

The temperature of the water is recommended to be around 29°C – assuming the workout is not too intense. Warmer water increases the elastic qualities of the muscles and helps to loosen the body, but it may also encourage milk flow from the breasts. Exercising in water that is too hot may cause the body to overheat and dehydrate. Water that is too cold will constrict blood vessels as the circulation is diverted away from the skin to maintain core temperature. Since the body cools down four times quicker in water than in air, appropriate planning of structure and content should be done to avoid mums standing still for too long.

Pool depth

The depth of the pool is relevant to both safety and effectiveness of exercise. Working out in chest-high water will support the joints, breasts and pelvic floor and significantly reduce the risk of injury and discomfort to these structures. It will also ensure a more effective workout than waist-high water by providing increased resistance to the upper body if the arms remain immersed. If positioned in waist-high water it is recommended to adopt a wide base and bend the knees in order to keep the breasts underwater.

When can you start?

Gentle swimming can be commenced when vaginal discharge has ceased – this may vary between three and five weeks after the birth. Other, more vigorous, water-based activities should not commence until a satisfactory postnatal check-up has been completed.

SHALLOW-WATER WORKOUT

Suitability

A shallow-water workout is done in water that is chest-high or less. This is a popular activity, performed to music, and is similar to a land-based exercise to music class, performed at a slower speed.

Considerations

Exercising in an appropriate depth of water is crucial to joint safety, breast comfort and exercise effectiveness. While chest-high water is preferable, a workout can be safely and effectively carried out in waist-high water if a wide leg base is adopted and the knees remain bent. Exercising in a group increases the turbulence of the water and adds a greater resistance to the workload. The stabilising muscles have to work much harder to maintain balance and consideration should be given to the degree of workload placed on the abdominal muscles in a supportive role. Strong rotational movements with the torso immersed should be avoided if the abdominal muscles remain separated.

Use simple, easy to follow movements that don't require too much co-ordination. Keep directional changes to a minimum and provide early cues when these are included. Use intervals to avoid overworking, by incorporating regular periods of rhythmical, flowing mobility movements. Avoid explosive movements out of the water. As a progression, and subject to good lumbopelvic stability, equipment such as webbed gloves, floats, buoys or bands may be used to increase the resistance.

DEEP-WATER WORKOUT

Suitability

Suitability of deep-water workouts

Deep-water workouts are not suitable for postnatal women. Due to the major role of the abdominal musculature in stabilising the body in deep water, participation should be postponed until lumbopelvic stability and abdominal group strength have been regained. Deep water is ideal for relaxation with the use of buoyancy aids.

SWIMMING

Suitability

Swimming is an excellent postnatal activity. It provides cardiovascular as well as local muscular benefits. Moderately paced swimming over a prolonged period of time will also utilise additional calories and help with weight loss. Gentle swimming can be particularly relaxing: the rhythmic action of the stroke, the feeling of weightlessness and the soft muffled sounds created by the water provide a calm, therapeutic quality not found in other activities.

Considerations

Despite the supporting effects of the water, any prone stroke performed with the head held high out of the water will increase compression of the cervical spine. This position causes the hips to sink and increases lumbar lordosis. Swimming in a head-down position realigns posture and allows the body to move more quickly through the water. Breaststroke leg action (in supine and prone) should be approached with caution for women recovering from PGP. A controlled ROM may help to loosen tight adductors and should be encouraged.

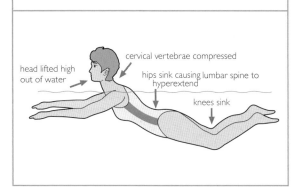

Figure 12.1 Incorrect swimming position

head lifted high out of water

cervical vertebrae compressed

hips sink causing lumbar spine to hyperextend

knees sink

SUMMARY

- Water workouts are particularly beneficial for joint and circulatory reasons.
- Stress to weight-bearing joints is greatly reduced.
- Body weight is reduced by 80 per cent when immersed to the chest.
- Body weight is reduced by 50 per cent when immersed to the waist.
- Water pressure stimulates the circulation and improves several postnatal conditions.
- Gentle swimming can commence as soon as discharge has ceased; more vigorous workouts should wait until after the postnatal check.
- Exercising the PFM in water is particularly helpful for muscular rehabilitation.
- Adequate breast support is essential – wearing a bra under the swimsuit is recommended.
- The breasts are at risk if they are not immersed – the knees should be bent to lower the body if exercising in waist-deep water.
- The abdominal muscles work hard to stabilise the body in water.
- Workload increases with turbulence and in deep water.
- Interval training is recommended to avoid overworking the abdominal muscles.
- Strong rotational movements should be avoided if the abdominal muscles are still separated.
- Intensity of workload is determined by the amount of effort used.
- Deep-water workouts should be postponed until lumbopelvic stability and abdominal group strength have been regained.
- Swimming provides excellent cardiovascular and local muscular benefits.
- Hyperextension of the cervical and lumbar spine may occur if the head is held too high out of the water.

RELAXATION

13

In addition to regular exercise, rest and relaxation should be an essential part of a new mum's lifestyle.

WHY IS RELAXATION SO IMPORTANT?

The arrival of a new baby places enormous physical and emotional demands on a woman, and unless adequate time is given to recharge her batteries she may experience mounting tension and fatigue, which could lead to stress.

STRESS

Stress is a threat to the body, either in the form of real danger, which requires immediate and fast reactions, or as a result of a series of problems and pressures that build up over a period of time. The body responds to stress by making various changes to prepare for the impending 'conflict'. Unfortunately we are unable to distinguish between real danger and emotional pressure, so if the situation or threat does not require a physical response, such as running away from danger, the body has no way of dispersing it. The continual presence of stressful situations demands the muscles be in a state of constant 'readiness', which is exhausting for the body.

Postnatal stress factors

Everyone is subjected to the stresses of everyday life, but a new baby brings additional physical and emotional pressures.

Physical factors

- Fatigue due to lack of sleep
- Sore, heavy breasts
- Sore perineum
- Constipation
- Pain or aching in the joints
- Muscular tension from postural changes
- Reduced energy levels

Emotional factors

- Being unable to settle baby
- Baby crying for long periods
- Concerns about the amount of feed baby is taking
- Having no time to do anything
- Inability to fit into normal clothes
- Feelings of loss of independence
- Feelings of inadequacy
- Feelings of isolation

What happens to the body under stress?

The body becomes aroused and this is reflected outwardly by postural changes:

- Head and body bent forwards
- Shoulders elevated
- Elbows bent and close to the body

- Fists clenched
- Legs crossed and ankles flexed (if seated)
- Jaw tightly shut and teeth clenched

Physiological changes also occur in response to stress: the heart rate, blood pressure and breathing rate increase; blood is diverted away from the skin and digestive system to the lungs and skeletal muscles ready for action; the mouth becomes dry; and sweating increases.

Once the situation has been dealt with, the body will return to normal with no harm done. If pressures continue, however, and the body is subjected to prolonged periods of arousal, the strain will begin to show, resulting in tension, frustration and fatigue.

Coping with stress

The first stage in dealing with stress is to recognise it. Pressures build up slowly, one on top of the other, and the body forgets how it feels to be calm and at ease. If the cause can be identified, the problems will be easier to deal with, but very often it is an accumulation of many factors, often minor, which soon escalate. Postnatal women may need reminding of their limitations, and have to be able to admit when they feel they can't cope.

TIME OUT AND RELAXATION

Taking time out is essential and, although she may feel it is inappropriate and self-indulgent, a mum should try to take the opportunity as often as possible. Her partner will probably enjoy the opportunity of spending time with baby without her watchful eye and, although copious instructions will be left, will probably manage very well! Taking up offers of assistance from others should be encouraged, as long as she understands that things may be done

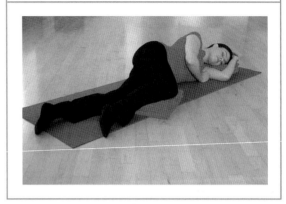

Figure 13.1 Relaxation

differently. Concerns over this may increase her anxiety, rather than making her feel relieved that the job has been done. Time off does not necessarily mean leaving the house; an allotted period of time at home, to spend as she chooses, may be an appropriate alternative. A period of relaxation is recommended.

Methods of relaxation

There are various methods of relaxation – the following three tend to be the most commonly used.

- **Contrast method:** This requires the individual contraction and release of all large muscle groups throughout the body. However, if the muscle is already feeling tense and tight, it is unable to let go and remains in a slightly contracted state.
- **Visualisation or imagery:** This involves the selection of a pleasant image, which stimulates positive thoughts and feelings. However, as this is mental imagery the physical state of the muscles is unaffected. There is also the possibility that an image may induce feelings of tension if bad experiences are visualised.
- **Physiological relaxation:** This method (also

known as the 'Mitchell Method') is widely taught during the antenatal period and, due to its simple exact technique, it is the most appropriate to continue into the postnatal period and beyond. It is based on the principle of reciprocal inhibition, i.e. muscles working in pairs – a muscle must relax to allow the opposing muscle to contract. The procedure and sequence of this method is explained below.

When is the best time for relaxation?

Whenever an appropriate opportunity arises is the simple answer! One could set time aside after a feed, when baby may sleep for a while; alternatively, if baby feeds well, it may be appropriate to attempt a short period of relaxation while breastfeeding, assuming there are no other children around to keep an eye on, or who may interrupt. Although this may not be as effective as relaxing alone, a comfortable, well-supported position will allow some degree of relaxation. Having learned the skill of relaxation, the body is able to let go much quicker. This means utilising more opportunities to switch off for five minutes at appropriate times during the day.

Where is the best place to relax?

Places where a comfortable position can be adopted are best – sitting at a table with head in hands, lying on the floor or bed, sitting up in a comfortable, supportive chair. A cushion or pillow can be placed under the head to support the neck, or under the thighs, if lying down, to make the back feel more comfortable.

Preparing to relax

It is important to wear warm, comfortable clothing without restriction. Cushions and pillows can be used for support as necessary and a blanket positioned nearby if required. Allow the body to sink into the support as you release yourself into position.

THE MITCHELL METHOD OF RELAXATION

This involves a set procedure of moving each joint into a position opposite to that of stress (*see* page 216 for examples), which encourages lengthening of the muscles that are causing tension. The instruction is then to 'stop' the movement and momentarily pause to consider how the new position feels. This gives the nerves time to register the change and makes it easier for the body to recall the position of ease again.

What position should be adopted?

Most benefit will be gained lying in a supine position, with cushions supporting the head and a small rolled up towel in the back if necessary. It can be done, however, in any comfortable, supported position but the instructions will need to be adapted.

Relaxation sequence

The method recommends that each joint is taken through the procedure in a fixed order as follows. The instructions are an individual variation of the original language used by Mitchell (1987).

Arms

Shoulders

- Pull the shoulders down, away from the ears
- Stop pulling
- Feel that the shoulders are lower and the neck longer

Elbows

- Move the elbows away from the body
- Stop moving
- Feel the elbows, open and away from the body

Hands

- Stretch out the fingers and thumbs
- Stop stretching
- Feel the hands, fingers and thumbs fully supported – be aware of the surface underneath the fingertips

Legs

Hips

- Roll the hips outwards
- Stop rolling
- Feel the legs slightly apart and rolled outwards

Knees

- Move the knees into a comfortable position
- Stop moving
- Be aware of the new position of the knees

Feet

- Flex the feet, drawing the toes towards the face
- Stop flexing
- Feel the feet hanging loosely from the ankles

Body

- Press the body into the support
- Stop pressing
- Feel the pressure of the body on the support

Head

- Press the head into the pillow/support
- Stop pressing
- Feel the head well-supported by the pillow

Face

Jaw

- Keeping the lips together, pull down the jaw
- Stop pulling
- Feel the teeth separated and the lips gently touching each other

Tongue

- Move the tongue to the middle of the mouth
- Stop moving
- Feel the tip of the tongue touching the lower teeth

Eyes

- Close the eyes (if not already closed)
- Be aware of the darkness

Forehead

- Raise the eyebrows towards the hairline
- Stop moving
- Feel the skin smoothing out and the hair moving

Breathing

- Take a deep breath in
- Feel the ribs moving outwards
- Breathe out easily

Once the sequence has been completed it can be repeated again a little faster, before remaining in the relaxed position for as long as circumstances permit.

Waking up

When the relaxation is over:

- Remain in position and open the eyes.
- Consider the new body positioning for a few seconds.
- Slowly rotate the wrists and then the ankles.
- Reach up above the head with the arms then release.

- Reach away from the hips with the legs then release.
- Reach up with the arms and away with the legs at the same time and release.
- Bend the knees up, one at a time, and place the feet flat on the floor.
- Roll carefully onto the side and rest there for a moment.
- When you feel ready to get up, slowly push yourself up with the hands and move into a sitting position.
- Lengthen the spine and sit tall.
- If time permits, remain in a comfortable seated position and perform the following remobilising moves.

Shoulder rolls

- Slowly circle one shoulder around in a large exaggerated way (forwards, upwards, backwards, downwards).
- Keep the spine long and the rest of the body still.
- Repeat as required.

Neck mobility

- Lengthen the spine and draw the shoulder blades down.
- Slowly take the head over to one side (ear to shoulder).
- Pause before returning to the upright position.
- Repeat as required.

Side bends

- Lengthen the spine.
- Bend slowly to the side, resting the hand on the floor for support.
- Return to the central position with the spine long.
- Repeat as required on alternate sides.

Spine mobility

- Round the back and slowly bring the shoulders and arms around in front at chest height.
- Lift and lengthen the body as the arms open to the side, drawing the shoulder blades down.
- Feel the chest opening and the spine lengthening.
- Draw the ribcage down to prevent the back from arching.
- Repeat as required.

Upward reach

- Place one hand on the floor beside the hip.
- Lift up through the body and reach up to the ceiling with the other arm.
- Keep the body weight slightly forwards.
- Lengthen through the side of the body.
- Lower the arm, keeping the body lifted and tall.
- Repeat on the other side.

Standing up

From the sitting position, move the body up to kneeling. Gently draw in the abdomen and drive up through the buttocks to a standing position (*see* Appendix for full details).

Time constraints of a full relaxation

If time and circumstances do not permit such a comprehensive relaxation on every occasion, this technique can be adapted for a shorter duration. The shortened version is ideal for use during a five-minute break in a comfortable chair.

Shortened version

Take the body through the same sequence, but use the end position of each body part as the only movement – this must be done slowly to allow time for the appropriate responses to occur. If the full relaxation technique is practised regularly, you should find that your body easily adopts the new positions.

Going through this sequence once a day will help release daily tensions and keep everything more manageable.

SUMMARY

- Relaxation is necessary to counteract the effects of stress.
- Physical and emotional factors increase muscular tension.
- Stress becomes exhausting for the body over a period of time.

- Time out and relaxation is essential for new mums.
- Women should be encouraged to be honest with themselves and admit when they can't cope.
- Take every opportunity to switch off for five minutes.
- Teach the body how to relax.

REFERENCE

Mitchell, L. 1987. *Simple Relaxation.* London, John Murray

PLANNING A POSTNATAL FITNESS SESSION

14

VENUE

The ideal venue should be easy to reach by public transport, with adequate car parking space close by. Buggy accessibility is important, with sufficient standing room within the exercise area, or other allocated storage space. Heating, lighting, ventilation, toilets etc. are essential. The facility should be clean and spacious (appropriate for the number of participants), free from obstacles and with a non-slip floor surface. Mats are essential for the floorwork sections.

PROMOTION

Contact with health professionals

The health visitor at the local clinic is an essential link with the postnatal community. She is the principal healthcare professional involved with new mums from approximately day 10 after delivery (the midwife may still be involved if there have been particular problems). The health visitor makes home visits to new mums and is responsible for the baby clinic at the local Health Centre/Children's Centre/GP surgery. Close liaison between the instructor and the health visitor could be extremely beneficial in increasing the advice available to postnatal women and creating an interest in specific postnatal exercise sessions. Through this source it may also be possible to visit postnatal groups by appointment, and to recommend and demonstrate appropriate exercises and back

care. This is an excellent method of professional promotion but it will be at the instructor's expense. Personal contact is extremely useful, as the majority of surgeries and clinics are not permitted to recommend services or hand out flyers.

Leaflets and posters

Subject to the relevant approval, these can be placed in a variety of locations: mother and toddler groups, playgroups, libraries, schools, shops, sports centres etc. Payment may be necessary.

Advertising

The NCT (National Childbirth Trust) is a very active organisation with branches all over the country. It is run predominantly by mums for mums and is an extremely successful network of support and advice for both antenatal and postnatal women. For a small fee, advertisements can be placed in branch newsletters, which are sent out quarterly to all members (branch details and contact numbers are usually available at the local library). The *Baby Directory*, a national publication published in regions, is available to purchase from leading bookshops. The *Parents' Directory*, also published in regions, is increasing its circulation around the UK and is distributed free through clinics, surgeries, and libraries (*see* Useful Contacts for more information).

Listings

Inclusion on the database listings provided by a library is another useful source of promotion. The library is an obvious public resource and the database holds information regarding class type, venue, day, time, contact number etc. This is also available online. Some local authorities publish an information book detailing facilities available for the under-fives in the area; activities for parents are also listed. Listings on websites such as Netmums are also useful.

SESSION ORGANISATION

An effective programme of postnatal exercise can really only be achieved by organising the sessions on a course basis (approximately 6–10 weeks in duration). Ideally, everyone begins together in week one and can then undergo a gentle introduction to exercise in a controlled and organised way. Sessions can progress in intensity and duration, with new exercises gradually introduced and practised, thus reducing the risk factors associated with irregular attendance. Different topics can be introduced and discussed each week to educate mums on PFM, abdominal recovery, lifting, carrying etc.

An advance booking system is recommended to avoid the difficulties of individuals just turning up for a session; this method ensures that all mums have been screened and follow-up enquiries made if necessary. Pre-payment also encourages commitment and regular attendance and improves results. This system requires a certain amount of administration to be successful.

Screening

Screening is essential to clarify suitability and identify specific contraindications or concerns. A postnatal screening form should establish the following:

- Date of delivery
- Type of delivery
- Episiotomy/stitches
- Breast/bottle feeding
- Date of postnatal check-up
- Result of postnatal check-up
- Joint or back problems
- Any other postnatal concerns
- Medical conditions
- Surgery in last two years
- Current medication
- Exercise history
- Allergies

Screening issues

Any issues arising should be discussed in confidence and participation only permitted if the instructor feels it is appropriate. *If in doubt, instructors should refer women back to their GP.* If conditions arise that the instructor is unfamiliar with, the woman should be asked for more details as she may have a good understanding of her condition. Instructors should make a point of doing further research as required, to be able to advise and guide women confidently in the future.

Do babies come along too?

Most women will need to bring their babies along with them. Crèche facilities may be provided in some venues but, because they are required to have a ratio of three babies to one carer, it is unlikely many babies can be accommodated. The only solution may be to bring the babies into the class and many women will prefer this anyway! Instructors working in clubs must gain permission from the management to ensure the venue has adequate insurance cover.

> ### Important!
>
> The presence of babies in an exercise setting has legal implications for the instructor; even though the mother is present, the instructor is still responsible for the safety and well-being of the baby in the class (Duty of Care clause within the Children's Act of 1996 – amended in 2004). This applies to any type of exercise session being conducted. Instructors must ensure that their insurance policy specifically stipulates that they are covered to teach classes where babies are present – if it doesn't check it out!

For the reasons of safety and well-being of the baby, it is essential in an indoor class that a 'baby zone' is created where the babies can be positioned away from the 'exercise zone'. *The babies do not enter the exercise zone and mums must not exercise in the baby zone.* This zone should be a clean space, not blocking access or fire exits, and free from hazards such as heaters, plug sockets and stacks of chairs.

In a buggy session the babies should remain in the buggy at all times while mum is exercising and she must stop exercising if baby comes out. It is the instructor's responsibility to ensure that babies are strapped in, when such straps are fitted, and tiny babies have adequate head support when travelling in a carry cot. Instructors must act responsibly and not include anything in the session that may increase the potential risk to babies, either directly or indirectly, e.g. running with the buggy, walking very close to water or positioning the buggy next to or underneath a potential hazard, such as a broken branch hanging from a tree.

A flexible teaching plan is essential with a group of unpredictable small babies, and instructors need to think on their feet and adapt as necessary.

Structure and content

A postnatal exercise session is structured to incorporate all the components of fitness. The following is applicable to all session types.

Warm-up

As well as warming, loosening and pulse-raising activities, this should include dynamic stretches.

Considerations

- Revise static and dynamic posture, taking into account the changes which have taken place in the body since delivery.
- Ensure controlled use of full range of movement during mobility.
- Use moderately paced pulse-raising activities.
- Incorporate dynamic stretching consisting of movements specific to the main workout which continue to warm and loosen.
- Encourage upright posture throughout.

CV

This should include a gradual rise in intensity, a short maintenance period and a gradual decline in intensity. Initially this should be a shallow curve, which becomes more defined (i.e. a sharper peak) as the course continues. The duration of the aerobic component may start with approximately 10 minutes and increase to 15–20 minutes over a 10-week period. There is insufficient time in a 60-minute class to do much more than this if adequate time is to be spent on the resistance component. The importance of the CV component should be explained, as some women may only be interested in lying on a mat and working their abdominals!

Considerations

- Use simple and easy to follow moves.
- Keep to low-impact activity.
- Perform sufficient repetitions to enable achievement.
- Keep to a moderate intensity – RPE of 4–6.

- Incorporate intermittent use of upper body work.
- Avoid fast knee-bending movements.
- Take care with long levers and momentum.
- If doing circuits, use standing stations to avoid mums having to go down to the floor and stand back up again at speed.
- Encourage upright posture throughout.

On completion of the CV component, if no further standing work is to be done, supported standing stretches may be included at this time for major muscle groups, particularly in the legs.

Resistance

In every session there should be a focus on the re-education of correct recruitment of deep stabilising muscles and time should be spent explaining how this is correctly performed. Many women will over-recruit and instructors must be patient and not feel pressurised to move on until everyone understands this.

Global muscle groups to be strengthened should include those:

- weakened by the effects of pregnancy (e.g. gluteus maximus/medius/minimus, lower trapezius);
- required for lifting, carrying and caring for baby (e.g. biceps, triceps, latissimus dorsi, quadriceps);
- which provide support for weakened joint structures (e.g. abductors, adductors, vastus medialis).

Considerations

- Advise a safe practice for getting down to the floor.
- Provide controlled and appropriate transitions.
- Suggest comfortable positions for breasts and pelvic floor.
- Include alternative positions and/or exercises where appropriate.

- Use an appropriate and effective pace.
- Make sensitive but effective use of sets and repetitions.
- Ensure controlled use of full range of movement where possible.

If this component is circuit-based, it should be taught as a command circuit, where all participants perform the same exercise at once. This provides a much more controlled environment when transitions, joint alignment and technique can be more effectively monitored. A multi-station circuit should only be taught when everyone is familiar with the movements – this is discussed under progression.

Cool-down

This should include stretches for all the muscle groups worked, a period of relaxation and a gentle wake-up.

Considerations

- Perform maintenance stretches only – no developmental stretches.
- Offer appropriate, comfortable positions for the individual.
- Provide alternative positions where appropriate, e.g. gluteal stretch and lying body reach for caesarean deliveries; some seated positions may be uncomfortable for those with a sore perineum.
- Comfortable stretches may be held for longer than 10 seconds, provided the range is not increased.
- Include a relaxation period. This is an essential part of the session and may be the only opportunity in the week for a new mum to rest and relax. There may not always be time to teach a full relaxation section, particularly towards the end of the course when the content is greater, but the opportunity to rest the body for a few minutes, with the inclusion of a few key relaxation points, will still be beneficial.

- Provide sufficient time for mums to wake up and refocus following a period of relaxation.

Progression

The following ideas for progression are suggested for a 6–10 week course:

Warm-up

The content of the warm-up may remain exactly the same from week to week. If the participants are new to exercise, it may take a few sessions to become familiar with the movements and to perform them correctly. Progression in this section is noticeable by a more effective performance of these movements. Instructors must remain focused on their client group and not switch to mainstream teaching mode by combining moves and introducing too much co-ordination, as that could reduce the quality and effectiveness of the work.

CV

Increasing duration is the main method of progression. Commence with approximately 10 minutes of aerobic work at the beginning of the course and increase it to about 15–20 minutes by the end, maintaining a moderate intensity. Movements should remain uncomplicated and easy to follow, as familiarity will improve performance and increase effectiveness. The curve of intensity may become more defined towards the end of the course, with a peak of slightly more intense activity in the middle of the component, although this would need to be carefully monitored. Depending on the ability of the group, the pace may increase slightly and arm work continue for longer than earlier in the course.

Resistance

The length of time spent on this section should stay the same, or may need to decrease slightly if more CV is included. However, more effective use of this time by quicker organisation and transitions and less rest allows additional exercises to be included and more sets to be performed. Intensity can also be increased by performing more repetitions, reducing the speed of the exercise or altering the body positioning to increase the resistance.

Towards the end of the course, when several muscle groups have already been introduced and need to be worked, there may be a tendency to rush through to include them all. While progression is important, the safe and correct performance of all exercises is essential and may result in some exercises, already taught, being omitted.

The use of a multi-station circuit could be included towards the end of the course but only if mums are familiar with all the exercises. Sufficient time should be allowed for getting into position, particularly if both standing and floor stations are being used: transitions from standing to floor and back up again should be taught and reminders given at every station.

Cool-down

Comfortable stretches should remain the same throughout the course and alternatives found where necessary. Although only maintenance stretches are included, some of the more passive positions could be held for slightly longer, provided no attempt is made to increase the range of movement.

It may be appropriate, as the course progresses, to extend the length of the relaxation as participants feel more able to relax and switch off. This will be dependent on whether babies are present and the total time available.

Due to the time constraints, instructors must be highly selective in their planning to enable progression to occur in all areas.

SUMMARY

- Venue location should be selected for easy access for all, including buggies.
- Advertising through a variety of mediums is recommended.
- The health visitor is the essential link with the postnatal community.
- Comprehensive screening is an essential part of professional care.
- Concerns should be referred back to the GP.
- Further research by the instructor may be required to accommodate individual problems.
- A course of fixed duration and organised attendance is recommended.
- If babies are present, they must be placed in a designated baby area and not enter the exercise area.
- In buggy workouts, babies must stay in their buggies throughout the session, or the mum must stop participating until baby has been safely returned – no exercises should be performed while holding baby.

- Even though the mum is present, instructors have a responsibility for the safety and well-being of the baby in the class.
- Instructors must ensure that their insurance policy specifically stipulates that they are covered to teach classes where babies are present.
- The structure and content of the session should consider the effects of pregnancy and delivery.
- Progression in all components of the session will help to improve physical fitness.

MANAGEMENT, TEACHING AND EVALUATION OF A POSTNATAL FITNESS SESSION

15

MANAGEMENT

In a fitness session, managing mums who are managing their babies can be *extremely challenging* even for the most experienced instructor.

The presence of their baby will be distracting for most mums, who will want to keep an eye on their little one. In an indoor exercise class, mums will frequently glance over to the baby zone; this lapse in focus will increase the risk of injury, particularly if mums are feeling tired. If babies become unsettled and mums have to leave the exercise area, it may be a few minutes before they return, at which point the class will have moved on to something else; mums will need to be refocused and additional guidance given. Frequent fussing over the babies will unsettle them and mums should be encouraged to leave them alone until their attention is really required.

Buggy workouts may allow mums to focus on the session a little more as the babies are with them; it is also easier to defuse a potential outburst while pushing a buggy. If babies become unsettled at stopping stations mums may be able to pacify them by pushing the buggy around and this is less disruptive to other mums and babies (and the instructor!). Buggy workouts do, however, require excellent group management skills, as working outdoors in a public place presents numerous surprises and potential hazards. Since the instructor is also responsible for the well-being of the baby, safety is paramount. An instructor must be able to respond to every situation that arises and maintain control and professionalism at all times.

TEACHING

Safe and effective teaching of this specialist group is determined by the demonstration of a series of practical skills, which highlight good practice. It is recommended that instructors develop these skills in the following sequential order, as achievement of the initial skills will enable successful application of the points that follow.

Organisation

Good organisation of the group will enable everyone to see and be seen and is an essential basic skill. Clear instructions should be given so mums know exactly where they should be positioned, and the use of arm movements to assist direction may be helpful. Make it clear whether they need to allow distance from their neighbours for a particular exercise. When using a wall for support, ensure that everyone is facing the same way; with floor work, be clear which way the mat should be arranged and which way the mum should be positioned on it. Good organisation will ensure that an appropriate teaching position can be adopted.

Teaching position

The instructor should be positioned to see and be seen by all participants in the group. This will involve a variety of positions during different sections of the session.

- Demonstrating movements from different angles provides a quick visual of the exercise and an opportunity to highlight areas of concern, e.g. turning the body sideways to reinforce spinal alignment.
- Leading a set of exercises with the back turned to the group may be helpful if the mirrored version is confusing to the participants. A brief demonstration in this position should be followed by the instructor turning to face the group so that group performance can be observed in the usual way.
- Turning the whole group around to face a different direction gives participants at the back an opportunity to see. It also allows the instructor to view individuals previously positioned behind others.
- Moving in the opposite direction to the group during a circle activity provides the opportunity for individual eye contact. Stepping out of the circle or circuit allows the instructor to scan the whole group.

Important!

Moving among the group while they continue a movement is essential. It provides an opportunity to observe posture, alignment and specific technique of individuals from a variety of angles.

The successful use of a variety of teaching positions is solely dependent on the initial organisation of the group. If, due to poor instructions, the participants face different directions, the position of the instructor will not be appropriate to everyone – this is particularly relevant during floorwork.

Demonstration

Excellent personal performance by the instructor is essential. The demonstration of correct postural alignment, accurate technique and clear, precise movements conveys very strong visual messages. Many people learn from watching so if the demonstration of the instructor is poor, the performance by the mums may be poor too. Movements should be strong, large and deliberate as this will motivate and encourage the use of effort; this is particularly relevant to upper body exercises, which often become weak and unclear. Only a few repetitions are necessary and they should be reinforced by a verbal explanation. Avoid having the group standing around watching – get them involved as soon as possible.

Explanation

Clear precise explanations are required without telling a story! Mums have come to exercise, not to listen to a long description of what they're going to be doing, so keep explanations brief and to the point. Explaining the purpose of the exercise is very beneficial; instructors are encouraged to educate mums as to what the exercise is for and how they will benefit from it. It is hoped this will increase their focus and may encourage home practice if an exercise is particularly relevant to their needs. Information should also be provided as to where exercises should be felt: as well as consolidating correct performance, this also draws the instructor's attention to individuals who are not experiencing sensation in the relevant area.

Explaining how to recruit TrA correctly will need to be recapped every session, and it may be necessary to discuss breathing techniques to avoid recruitment of the global stabilisers (*see* chapter 2). The PFM will need similar attention: structure, function and recruitment should be clearly explained in detail in the first session, and correct recruitment reinforced in later sessions. Instructors should use friendly language, appropriate to the group.

Teaching points

Teaching points are vital to ensure both the safety and the effectiveness of the exercise. A range of points should be used to make sure that movements are performed in a safe and appropriate way. These should be relevant to the technique of each movement, with particular concern for joint alignment and the maintenance of correct posture. Reinforcement of the essential points must continue for the duration of the movement and be reiterated in each session.

Teaching points should be delivered as short, clear statements focusing on the positive, preventative care necessary to avoid a problem occurring. Pacing the delivery, rather than gushing forth with a whole host of points that cannot be utilised, allows points to be processed. Recurring points may be given in a variety of ways to maintain interest. When new exercises are introduced, teaching points should be delivered one at a time, continuing only when the previous one has been achieved.

As awareness and skill develop, so the focus should change from safety to effectiveness, but still with safety in mind. It is vital that the use of these valuable points is accompanied by correct technical performance by the instructor.

Voice

The voice should be clear and audible throughout the session, and delivered at an appropriate pace to enable participants to process the infor-mation and react accordingly. Tone, volume and mood should be varied according to the component being taught. Tone and volume may also change as the participants become more able: a gentle, persuasive approach to the initial sessions may develop to a much more dynamic, motivating style as the course progresses. Sensitivity and encouragement must be shown at all stages of a postnatal course.

Teaching outdoors puts extra demands on the voice. Not only does the instructor have to project into an open space, but there is also the noise of others around, together with wind and rain, to contend with on occasions.

Observation

Good observation skills are vital, predominantly for safety but also for movement effectiveness. Instructors must get out into the group and move around as soon as possible so that individual performance can be observed and corrected as necessary. The ability to look at the performance of the group and pick out individual problems is an essential and invaluable skill, and involves close scrutiny of posture and joint alignment, particularly when speed and intensity increase. This can be done by first scanning the group for problems before homing in on any safety issues picked up. Working methodically along a line of mums increases the risk of poor performance continuing for longer, so the instructor must be pro-active and move around as soon as possible. Working outdoors when mums are wearing several layers of clothing may make it more difficult to observe form. *Standing still in front of the group or performing exercises with them is unprofessional and inappropriate.*

Movements are extremely difficult to observe if only a few repetitions are performed and the choreography is complex. Careful planning is important to ensure that combinations are repeated sufficiently to allow effective observation. As well as observing technical performance, it is also important to make eye contact. This shows concern for the individual, not just for the body being moved, and helps to build confidence and rapport; it also encourages a more effective performance. Indications of fatigue and strain can be seen in facial expressions as well as the satisfied smiles of enjoyment and achievement.

Technically correct but ineffective performance requires a higher level of skill to recognise, but this is another vital element to successful teaching. Once participants become familiar with the content of the session, their performance must be carefully monitored for the degree of effort used.

Having observed performance, instructors must provide appropriate feedback as required.

Feedback

There are three types of feedback:
- Correction of inappropriate technique, speed or intensity
- Improvement of ineffective performance
- Praise and encouragement

Poor technique must be corrected immediately to prevent damage to the vulnerable joints and muscles. It may be necessary to make immediate eye contact while offering the correction, to ensure that the individual is aware of the level of concern. This can be reinforced if the teaching position is changed and the correct method demonstrated, highlighting alignment from a different angle. If this does not have the desired effect, it may be necessary to move alongside or immediately in front of the individual. Correct technique should then be reinforced every time this movement occurs during the session and should be reiterated in the following weeks.

Giving feedback to improve performance is essential if exercise is to be beneficial. A lack of appropriate feedback often results in little effort being used, and although the moves are performed safely, they are ineffective. The instructor must work hard to ensure that individuals are putting sufficient effort into the movements and extending, bending, pushing, and pulling in the most effective but safest way. A more dynamic use of voice and body language is often very helpful. Additional demonstrations by the instructor of a more effective performance should assist.

Praise and encouragement are essential in this rather technically oriented session. Positive feedback to participants will motivate, encourage better performance and, above all, increase self-confidence.

Adaptations and alternatives

These may be necessary for the following reasons:
- Discomfort experienced in the required position/movement
- Tiredness
- Inappropriate intensity

A range of levels should be demonstrated in all components whenever possible, so that participants can choose the appropriate level for themselves for that day. Options for varying levels of arm work during an aerobic component and a choice of body positions for press-ups, for example, are both relevant general alternatives, which can be offered to everyone. Specific adaptations for individual conditions should, where possible, involve the same muscle group, although if a similar body position is required it may still be inappropriate. If the position itself is causing the problem, an alternative exercise may need to be given in another position. PFME can be performed in any position.

Once again, if the session is to be effective, the level of intensity selected by individuals should be appropriate to their ability; very often the easiest option will be taken by individuals who can obviously cope with more. It is up to the instructor to educate the group about exercise effectiveness and encourage awareness of full performance as often as possible. There will be occasions when this degree of effort is not possible: these should be dealt with sensitively.

Session evaluation

Evaluation plays a crucial role in professional development, yet unfortunately it is often a neglected part of teaching. Reflecting on a session previously taught will allow the instructor to identify areas for improvement. The following questions provide an idea of the depth of information necessary to make a comprehensive evaluation.

CHECKLIST FOR STRUCTURE AND CONTENT

In the warm-up did you...

- Warm and loosen the joints through the normal ROM?
- Consider joint alignment?
- Use the warm-up to prepare the body for the main event?
- Incorporate moves which could be unsafe?

In the CV component did you...

- Plan a graduated curve of intensity?
- Induce breathing and heart rate changes?
- Encourage feedback regarding intensity and adapt accordingly?
- Consider the degree of impact and stress to joints, breasts and PFM?
- Consider joint alignment?
- Use appropriately paced movements?

- Include easy to follow movements?
- Include any movements which could be unsafe?

In the resistance component did you...

- Spend sufficient time focusing on correct recruitment of deep stabilising muscles?
- Include PFME in isolation?
- Select appropriate muscle groups for postural correction?
- Provide sufficient resistance and repetitions to make these effective?
- Consider joint alignment?
- Use appropriately paced movements?
- Include any exercises which could be unsafe?
- Provide safe transitions between exercises?

In the cool-down did you...

- Stretch all muscles worked?
- Stretch other muscles affected by pregnancy postural changes?
- Consider joint alignment?
- Provide safe transitions between exercises?
- Provide a short period for rest and/or relaxation?
- Provide appropriate wake-up exercises?

How can you improve the structure and content of your session?

CHECKLIST FOR TEACHING

Organisation – did you...

- Clearly direct the group into position?
- Make certain that everyone was facing the correct way?
- Ensure that everyone had sufficient space to exercise effectively?

Teaching position – did you...

- Use it to emphasise postural alignment?

- Vary it to demonstrate movements?
- Move around the group to observe all the participants?

Demonstration – did you...

- Perform with correct alignment?
- Demonstrate in a strong, dynamic way?
- Participate in the session with the group?

Explanations – did you...

- Use clear and precise instructions?
- Explain the purpose of the exercises?
- Tell the group where the exercise should be felt?
- Educate the group?

Teaching points – did you...

- Give teaching points appropriate to the content?
- Emphasise posture and exercise safety?
- Provide sufficient teaching points?
- Reinforce teaching points?
- Use a variety of terms to say the same thing?
- Deliver the points at an appropriate pace?
- Deliver points clearly and precisely?

Voice – did you...

- Speak clearly and audibly?
- Vary your tone and volume according to the components?
- Show sensitivity to your client group?
- Motivate and encourage?

Observation – did you...

- Move around the group?
- Observe incorrect technique?
- Observe ineffective performance?
- Make eye contact?
- Observe facial expressions?

Feedback – did you...

- Correct inappropriate technique?
- Improve individual performance?

- Reinforce teaching points?
- Improve ineffective performance?
- Encourage more effort from everyone?
- Encourage more effort from individuals?
- Praise effort and good performance?

Adaptations and alternatives – did you...

- Offer a range of levels?
- Demonstrate all options?
- Offer alternative positions?
- Teach the alternative positions?
- Observe the alternative positions?

How can you improve your teaching?

Did the participants...

- Enjoy the session?
- Feel they had an effective workout?
- Express a desire to come again?
- Provide any additional feedback?

SUMMARY

- Managing mums with babies present in the class can be very challenging.
- Mums will be easily distracted and their attention needs to be refocused.
- The safety of mother and baby is paramount.
- Advanced teaching skills are required to teach this specialist group.
- Good practice is achieved by a series of competencies.
- Organisation of the group is essential, to see and be seen.
- Teaching position should vary according to the activity.
- The personal performance of the instructor should be strong, precise and correct.
- Explanations should be clear and precise and employ user-friendly language.
- Teaching points relate primarily to the safety of the movements, and secondarily to their effectiveness.

Figure 1 Safe transition from standing to supine lying

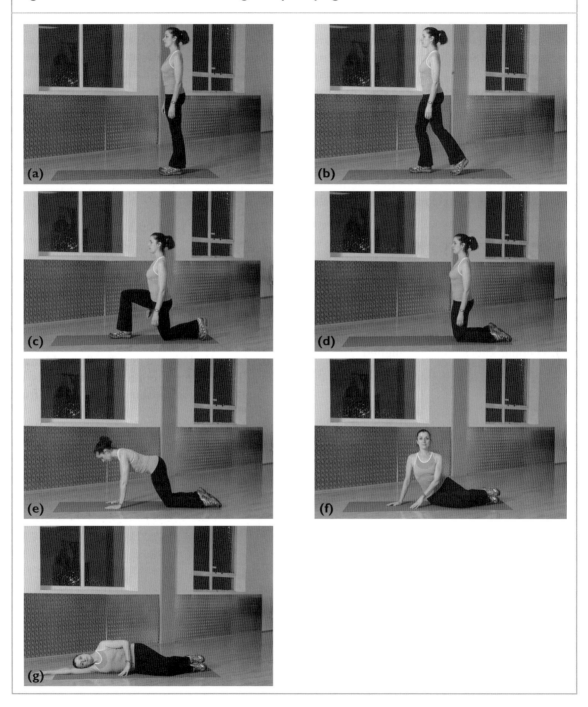

LIFESTYLE ADVICE

Getting in and out of bed

- Sit on the edge of the bed, with feet flat on the floor.
- Lie down onto the side and lift legs onto the bed.
- Moving the whole body together, gently turn over onto the back, keeping knees and feet aligned.
- Reverse the process when getting out of bed.
- Avoid coming straight to a sitting position from lying down, as this stresses the abdominal muscles and spine.

Sitting up from lying down in the bath

If possible, roll over to the side as before. However, if space is limited recruit TrA before using arms to push up to sitting.

Standing while holding baby

When standing with baby on one shoulder, there may be a tendency to lean slightly backwards to keep the baby in position – particularly when it is very small and has no head control. If this is practised for long periods at a time, the lumbar spine becomes stressed in this overextended position, which may induce backache. Be sure to stand in correct postural alignment with the spine in neutral and draw the ribcage down. Straddling the baby across

Figure 2 Standing while holding baby (a) Incorrect posture – straddling baby across hip (b) Correct posture

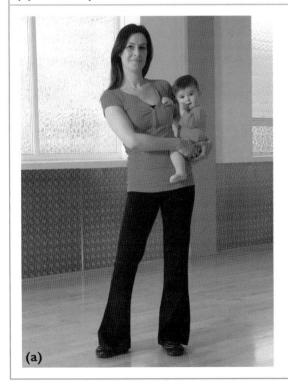
(a)

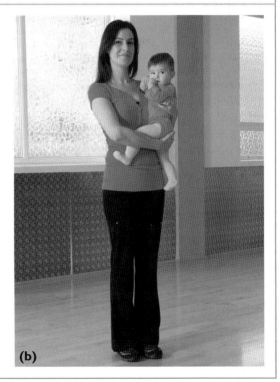
(b)

one hip lifts the hip, distorts spinal alignment and causes uneven pressure on the SP/SIJ. Keeping the hips in line does not provide as much support for the baby but is much safer for the pelvis.

Feeding posture

Whether breast or bottle feeding, the adopted seated position is just as important as when standing, as many hours may be spent there! Sitting in a slumped position switches off the deep stabilising muscles, which could have been working away while feeding. Rounding forwards over baby also causes back and neck ache. The following guidelines should be observed:

- Select a chair on which upright posture can be adopted – a very soft, bucket-shaped seat is inappropriate.
- Sit back into the chair so the spine is supported.
- Place cushions in the small of the back and sit tall.
- Place feet on a footstool or pile of books, to raise the height of the knees.
- Lie baby on a pillow to bring him closer.

Maintaining correct seated posture may be extremely hard, particularly if breastfeeding is proving difficult. Poor feeding positions may be held for some time if baby has problems latching on to the breast and it is feared that changing the position may disrupt the feed. Try to avoid them if possible.

Bathing baby

Lifting and lowering a heavy baby bath full of water should be avoided at all costs. Choose a baby bath that rests over the main bath so you can fill and empty it in situ, and kneel alongside to bath the baby. Alternatively, use the bathroom basin when baby is small. Bath seats are ideal for older babies.

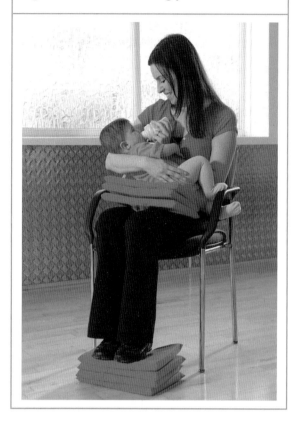

Figure 3 Correct feeding posture

Changing baby

- Use a work surface that is at waist height, if possible, to prevent stooping.
- Alternatively, kneel at the side of the bed, although this may become very demanding on the knees.
- Position all the equipment in front or to the side to prevent twisting behind.

Carrying baby

If carrying baby for any length of time, it is much better to use a baby sling worn at the front and positioned as high as possible to avoid leaning back. When carrying shopping, try to distribute the weight evenly between the bags and be sure

Figure 4 Bending and lifting baby

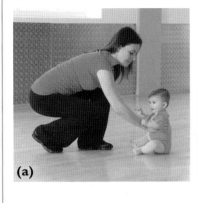
(a)

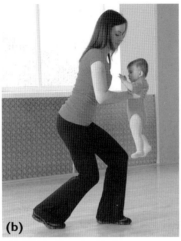
(b)

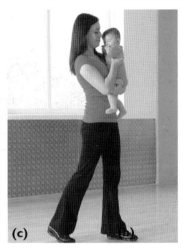
(c)

to recruit TrA when bending to pick up or put down. Alternatively, use a backpack.

Bending and lifting baby

The curtsey lunge on page 110 is designed to train mums to bend and lift correctly.

Stand in a shortened split stance, with correct upright posture. Recruit TrA and lift the back heel off the floor, bending both knees and hinging forwards from the hips. Lower the buttocks towards the heel of the back foot, reaching the arms towards the floor in front to take hold of baby. Tighten the PFM and gluteals and drive up to standing using the buttocks, at the same time moving baby in towards the body. Maintain natural breathing.

RATE OF PERCEIVED EXERTION

This is a subjective method of assessing exercise intensity, by rating the degree of physical exertion an individual is feeling. It is measured against the scale below for a reading between 1 and 10. The recommended intensity for postnatal mums is between 4 and 6.

The scale in table 1 is adapted from the revised Borg Scale of Perceived Exertion.

Table 1	Scale of perceived exertion
Perceived exertion	**Scale**
No exertion at all / relaxed	0
Very, very light / no problem	1
Very light / very easy	2
Fairly light / easy	3
Moderate / beginning to feel puffed	4
Fairly hard / feeling a bit puffed	5
Hard / feeling puffed	6
Very hard / tiring	7
Very, very hard / very tiring	8
Exhausted / out of breath / shattered	9
Maximum / exhausted	10

GLOSSARY

Acetabulum – cup-shaped socket which receives the head of the femur.

Actin – one of two proteins (along with myosin) responsible for muscular contraction.

Active stretch – using another muscle in order to achieve a stretch (e.g. when the body is actively involved in holding a stretch).

Adductors – gluteus medius and minimus muscles.

Adductors – the muscles of the inner thigh.

ADL – activities of daily living.

Amenorrhoea – cessation of menstruation (periods).

Aponeurosis (abdominal) – a sheet-like, tendinous expansion connecting the abdominal musculature to the linea alba.

ASIS (anterior superior iliac spines) – bony points at the front of the iliac crest.

Atrophy – decrease in muscle mass.

Cadence – the number of steps per minute or the stride rate.

Cantilever buggy – a stroller-type buggy with hook-shaped handles.

Carpal tunnel syndrome – a condition, associated with water retention, where compression of the median nerve in the wrist causes tingling and numbness in the thumb and the index and middle fingers.

Cartilaginous joint – connected by cartilage.

Coccyx – four fused vertebrae joined to the sacrum, often referred to as the tailbone.

Cervical vertebrae – seven vertebrae in the neck.

Closed chain exercise – working a limb which is anchored so that the joints move in a predetermined way.

Collagen – the main component of connective tissue.

Colostrum – a yellowish fluid produced by the breasts during pregnancy and the first few days after delivery.

Concentric contraction – the muscle shortens as it contracts.

Connective tissue – binds together and supports body structures (e.g. tendons, ligaments, cartilage and fascia).

Corpus luteum – the outer covering of the ovarian follicle, left behind after ovulation.

Decidua – the lining of the pregnant uterus.

Deltoids – the muscles covering the tops of the shoulders.

Denervation – loss of nerve supply.

Developmental stretching – stretching to increase the range of movement.

Diaphragm – the muscular partition between the abdominal and thoracic cavities.

Diastasis recti – separation of the recti muscles.

Doming – a bulge in the abdominal wall occurring during contraction of rectus abdominis when the muscles are still separated.

Eccentric contraction – the muscle lengthens as it contracts.

Facet joints – the joints of the articular processes of two adjacent vertebrae.

Fascia – connective tissue separating muscle layers and encasing them in a sheath.

FITT – Frequency, Intensity, Time and Type – the method used to increase fitness.

Fixator muscle – the muscle which stabilises the joint to prevent unnecessary movements while the prime mover is contracting.

Flexibility training – movements that increase the range of movements at a joint.

Gait – the pattern of the limbs during movement.

Gastrocnemius – the large muscle in the calf.

Gluteals – a group of muscles which cover the hip joint and much of the pelvis.

Gluteus medius/minimus – a group of muscles attaching onto the side and back of the pelvis, known collectively as the abductors.

Gluteus maximus – the largest muscle of the gluteal group, commonly referred to as the buttocks.

Haemorrhoids – varicose veins of the anus.

Hip flexors – the muscles connecting the lower spine and pelvis to the top of the femur.

Hydrostatic pressure – the pressure exerted by water on the tissues of the body when immersed.

Hyperextension – overextending a joint.

IAP (intra-abdominal pressure) – pressure created by the synchronised contraction of TrA, diaphragm, PFM and multifidus to provide spinal support.

Ilium – the wing-shaped bone of the pelvis.

Iliopsoas – group of muscles referred to as the hip flexors.

Inner range training – method used to shorten a muscle which has lengthened as a result of postural changes (e.g. RA, where the muscle is required to hold a contraction at the innermost range).

Interdigitate – to interlock like fingers.

Ischial tuberosities – the sitting bones.

Ischium – the thick, lower part of the pelvis leading down to the ischial tuberosities.

Isometric – muscular contraction where the muscle stays the same length (static contraction).

Isotonic – muscular contraction where the muscle changes length (concentric or eccentric).

Knack – the counter-contraction of the PFM prior to loading (e.g. when coughing, sneezing or lifting).

Kyphosis – outward curvature of the thoracic spine and sacrum.

Lactation – period of time relating to milk production.

Lateral rotation – turning outwards, also known as external rotation.

Latissimus dorsi – the broad muscle in the middle and lower back.

Levator ani – the deep muscles of the pelvic floor.

Ligaments – connective tissue supporting the joints and organs.

Linea alba – a tendinous band situated down the mid-line of the abdomen, formed by the joining of the aponeuroses of the abdominal muscles.

Lordosis – exaggerated inward curvature of the lumbar or cervical spine.

Lumbar vertebrae – five vertebrae of the lower back.

Maintenance stretching – stretches to maintain range of movement where the position of tension is held but not extended.

Mastitis – an inflammation of the breast tissue when milk is not emptied as quickly as it is produced.

Medial rotation – turning inwards, also known as internal rotation.

Multifidus – a deep spinal muscle activated with TrA to provide lumbopelvic stability.

Multiparity – the condition of having had more than one child.

Mobility – movement of a joint within its natural range.

Myosin – one of two proteins (along with actin) responsible for muscular contraction.

Neutral spine – the natural, correct alignment of the spine, which allows the body systems to function at their optimum level.

Oestrogen – a female hormone, essential for the menstrual cycle, produced in large quantities during pregnancy, when it is associated with the growth of the baby.

Obliques – two layers of abdominal muscle, the internal and external obliques, which are responsible for flexion and rotation of the trunk.

Open chain exercise – working a limb which is free to move in any direction.

Overload – placing greater demands on the body than it is accustomed to.

Passive stretch – when an external force, such as gravity or a partner, is involved in achieving a stretch.

Parallel – both feet aligned, facing forwards.

Patella – the knee cap.

Pectoral muscles – the muscles of the chest.

Perineum – the area between the anus and the vagina.

PF (pelvic floor) – a muscular platform at the base of the pelvis.

PFM (pelvic floor muscles) – the key players in lumbopelvic stability, forming part of the inner unit of stabilising muscles.

PGP – pelvic girdle pain.

Piriformis – a deep external rotator of the hip.

Prime mover – the key muscles responsible for joint action.

Principles of training – Frequency, Intensity, Time and Type – the method used to improve fitness.

Prolactin – the hormone responsible for stimulating milk production.

Prolapse – bulging of the bladder or rectum into the wall of the vagina, or the descent of the uterus into the vagina.

Progesterone – a female hormone, essential to the menstrual cycle, produced in large quantities during pregnancy, when it is responsible for relaxing smooth muscle tissue.

Prone – front lying.

Proprioception – the body's sense of position in response to a stimuli.

PSIS (posterior superior iliac spines) – bony points at the back of the iliac crest.

Pudendal nerve – responsible for activating the pelvic floor muscles.

Pubis – bone situated at the front of the pelvis.

Q angle – the angle of the femur from the hip to the knee.

RA (rectus abdominis) – the two bands of abdominal muscles which run down the centre of the abdomen and undergo tremendous stretching and separation during pregnancy.

Raphe – the unison of two symmetrical structures (e.g. linea alba).

Rec check – procedure for checking the width of separation of the bands of rectus abdominis.

Reciprocal inhibition – the process of a muscle relaxing in order that the opposing muscle can contract.

Relaxin – a hormone, produced in larger amounts during pregnancy, which increases connective tissue elasticity and reduces joint stability.

Resorption – process by which a structure is remodelled.

ROM – range of movement of a joint.

RPE (rate of perceived exertion) – a subjective method of assessing how hard the body is working.

Sacrum – triangular-shaped bone made up of five fused vertebrae.

Sarcomere – the contractile unit of the muscle.

Sciatica – pain in the buttock which may radiate down the back of the leg.

SIJ (sacroiliac joints) – two joints at the back of the pelvis formed by the unity of the ilium and the sacrum.

Sphincter – ring of muscle that contracts to close an opening.

Soleus – deep muscle of the calf.

SP (Symphysis pubis) – the joint at the front of the pelvis joining the two pubic bones together.

Split stance – standing with one foot in front of the other, hip-width apart.

Stretch weakness – changes occurring in muscles which have undergone adaptive lengthening as a result of postural changes.

Supine – back lying.

Thoracic spine – the 12 vertebrae in the mid-section of the back.

Toeing out – standing with the feet turned out at '10 to 2'.

TrA (transversus abdominis) – the deepest abdominal muscle, responsible for compression of the abdominal wall and for lumbar spine stabilisation.

Training effect – physiological adaptations of the body as a result of overload.

Trapezius – triangular-shaped muscle in the neck and upper back.

Umbilicus – the navel.

Valley cushion – an inflatable cushion with a gulley down the centre, used to provide a comfortable sitting position for women with perineal or coccyx discomfort.

Valsalva manoeuvre – the action of forced exhalation through a closed airway to increase intra-thoracic pressure.

Varicose veins – swollen veins with ineffective valves which are unable to close and secure one-way flow of blood.

Vastus medialis – a muscle of the quadriceps group specifically responsible for the last 15 degrees of knee extension.

Venous return – the flow of blood back to the heart.

Xiphisternum – the tip of the sternum.

RECOMMENDED READING

Behnke, R.S. 2001. *Kinetic Anatomy.* Leeds: Human Kinetics

Byrne, H. 2001. *Exercise after Pregnancy.* Berkeley: Celestial Arts

Calais-Germain, B. 1993. *Anatomy of Movement.* Seattle: Eastland Press Inc.

Creager, C. 1996. *Therapeutic Exercises Using Foam Rollers.* Berthoud: Executive Physical Therapy Inc.

Creager, C. 1998. *Therapeutic Exercises Using Resistance Bands.* Berthoud: Executive Physical Therapy Inc.

Creager, C. 2001. *Bounce Back Into Shape After Baby.* Berthoud: Executive Physical Therapy Inc.

Lawrence, D. 1998. *Complete Guide to Exercise in Water.* London: A & C Black

Lee, D. 2007. *The Pelvic Girdle.* Oxford: Churchill Livingstone

Mantle, J., Haslem, J. & Barton, S. 2004. *Physiotherapy in Obstetrics and Gynaecology.* Oxford: Butterworth-Heinemann

Mitchell, L. 1987. *Simple Relaxation.* London: John Murray

Norris, C.M. 2000. *Back Stability.* Leeds: Human Kinetics

O'Dwyer, M. 2009. *Hold It Sister: The Confident Girl's Guide to a Leak-free Life.* Queensland, Australia: Redsok

Patel, K. 2005. *Corrective Exercise: A Practical Approach.* London: Hodder Arnold

Paterson, J. 2009. *Teaching Pilates for Postural Faults, Illness and Injury.* Oxford: Butterworth-Heinemann

Porter, S. (ed.) 2008. *Tidy's Physiotherapy* 14th edn. Oxford: Churchill Livingstone

Robinson, L., Fisher, H., Knox, J. & Thomson, G. 2000. *Official Body Control Pilates Manual.* London: Macmillan

Sapsford, R.R., Bullock-Saxton, J. & Markwell, S.J. 1999. *Women's Health: A Textbook for Physiotherapists.* London: Saunders

USEFUL CONTACTS

ADVERTISING

www.netmums.com
www.babydirectory.com
www.nctpregnancyandbabycare.com
www.parentsdirectories.com

INSTRUCTOR TRAINING

Pushy Mothers

A company offering buggy workouts to post-natal mums, instructor training for the Pushy Mothers training systems and antenatal/post-natal exercise training for health professionals. All courses are accredited by the Royal College of Midwives, and the buggy workout training has received a commendation from the Association of Chartered Physiotherapists in Women's Health.
www.pushymothers.com

The Guild of Pregnancy and Postnatal Exercise Instructors

An organisation offering study days for qualified antenatal/postnatal fitness instructors.
www.postnatalexercise.co.uk

PGP SUPPORT GROUPS

www.pelvicpartnership.org.uk
www.pelvicinstability.org.uk

POSTNATAL DEPRESSION

www.rcpsych.ac.uk
www.beyondblue.org.au
www.pni.org.uk
www.mama.co.uk

INDEX